BABYLOVE

When lovers change into parents what happens to their loving? Pregnancy does not have to mean the end of a satisfying sex life as many people think. In fact, it can be the most loving, tender, sensuous time of your life. And this book tells you *exactly* how.

BabyLove mums have a relaxed attitude to mothering which means that babycare is never a wearying grind for them. They would rather be champion cuddlers than first rate cleaners. What does it matter if nappies go grey in the wash as long as they're pinned on a smooth, healthy bottom? BabyLove mums know that all you need to be a successful mum is love. Dads will also find lots to involve them in this book. When a couple truly share the responsibility of a child the work is halved and the love doubled. As some famous fathers including Paul McCartney, Sylvester Stallone and Donald Sutherland explain inside.

BabyLove is the first and only *fun* guide to pregnancy and loving parenthood through the first wonderful year of your child's life.

ABOUT THE AUTHORS

Val Hudson and Judy Wade are both national
newspaper journalists. They met when
employed on the women's pages of *The Sun*
newspaper.
Both writers were featured in *The Sun* when their
first babies were born in 1975. Val Hudson
wrote a series of articles before she conceived
and throughout her pregnancy on the subject
of becoming a mum. She also appeared
throughout her pregnancy on B.B.C.1's popular
programme *Pebble Mill* talking to, among
others, doctors, geneticists and sex-diviners
about the various stages of pregnancy.
Judy Wade had her baby by acupuncture, only
the second mother in Britain to use this method
of pain relief. Both authors had their babies
after an induced birth. Val had the epidural
form of anaesthetic after seven hours of natural
childbirth, and both had episiotomies (a cut in
the pelvic wall).
Their experiences are the basis of this book.
Both authors have lived in Britain for many
years but were born abroad, Judy in Australia,
Val in South Africa. With their journalistic
experience and their experience as new mums
aided by a panel of medical experts they feel
their book is packed, not just with *all* the
medical know-how you need, but also with a
lot of lively, amusing anecdotes proving that
pregnancy and parenthood can be *fun*!

BabyLove

A practical guide to a loving pregnancy and parenthood

Judy Wade and Val Hudson

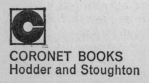

CORONET BOOKS
Hodder and Stoughton

FOR OUR MOTHERS, OUR DAUGHTERS AND
THE MEN WHO MADE US MOTHERS

First published in Great Britain 1977 by
Coronet Books
Second impression 1977

Printed and bound in Great Britain for
Hodder and Stoughton Paperbacks, a
division of Hodder and Stoughton Ltd.,
Mill Road, Dunton Green, Sevenoaks,
Kent (Editorial Office: 47 Bedford
Square, London, WC1 3DP), by
Hunt Barnard Printing Ltd.,
Aylesbury, Bucks.

ISBN 0 340 21977 7

Acknowledgments

This book would still be just a gleam in our eyes if it weren't for the inspiration and information gained from the following:

Gynaecologist Dr. Rosamond Bischoff; G.P. Sheila Fletcher; health visitor Jean Minty; chief medical adviser to the Wellcome Foundation U.K. Dr. William Currie; midwife Ann Latchford; editor of *Nursery World* Penny Kitchen; obstetric physiotherapist Margie Polden; psychologist Dr. Sam Baxter; psychologist Jane Firbank; psychiatric social worker, Betty Eve; journalist Jean Ritchie, Sue Snell and Camilla Sorsbie; B.B.C. T.V. Further Education producer Peter Riding; a Department of Health and Social Security civil servant; Queen Charlotte's Maternity Hospital, the Elizabeth Garrett Anderson Hospital and the Royal Free Hospital; also the countless mums who gave us their experiences and tips, especially Joyce, Angela, Barbara, Roslyn, Patsy, Yael, Heather, Yvette and Annie.

Our special thanks to the ladies who toiled with our kids while we typed: Madge Newton, Lyn McConnell, Sue and Fiona Geraghty, Sharon and Shirley Clover, Louise Smith and Joan de Peyer.

Contents

Bottle feeding:
  Choosing a milk
  Equipment
  How to start
  Making up feeds
  How to bottle feed
  Other drinks. Vitamins
  Is the baby still hungry?
  Is burping necessary

An Introduction by the Authors' Husbands

We would like to thank Val and Judy for making us fathers. It was a pleasure making them mothers. But not long after they had produced our dazzling daughters, they decided to give birth to this book. We asked them why – after all, there are dozens of baby books on the market. So they told us: that although other books tell mums how to cope with the responsibilities and problems of pregnancy, there isn't one which also explains that becoming a mum can be *fun*. In fact, the most loving, lovely time of a girl's life. They wanted to write a book reminding women that it still takes two to make a baby because father is too often the forgotten partner in the team job of making and bringing up a baby. Food to find and dragons to slay can mean that fathers are left out of a baby's life or get pushed into the background in the explosion of nappies and noise that follows the end of a pregnancy.

We agree when they say that if fathers are not really involved with their babies from the start, it's not good for the babies – or the fathers. But that doesn't mean that a baby should be king or queen of the household. (Incidentally, in this book, the baby is always referred to as 'she', not just because we have daughters but because all those other books always call the baby 'he'.)

There's another aspect that most other baby books forget, too – that mothers should always be lovers, too. Sex is *not* the most important part of a marriage, except when it goes wrong. And it can go wrong if loving lapses when a baby is on the way. Once stopped, it's hard to restart. Well, this book tells you how to have a sexy pregnancy – with illustrations to show you *exactly* how (*see* chapter six). It proves that sex during pregnancy isn't risky but the best way to produce both happy parents and healthy babies. So you see, this book is a kind of combination of the Kama Sutra and a babycare manual!

Producing *BabyLove* meant a lot more late meals and preoccupied wives and even more fuss than it takes to produce a baby. But we think the effort was worth while. Without it, we might not have been left holding the baby so often and discovered that little girls learn to flirt much younger than we suspected!

Robin and Vincent.

CHAPTER ONE

A Loving Start

Pregnancy starts and ends in bed. It usually begins with sweet passion on the bouncy innerspring at home. But too often it ends with an exhausting ordeal on a high hospital bed in a world of masked strangers, hard lights and cold machines. So the belief grows that making babies is lovely – but having them isn't.

We believe it doesn't have to be like that. Childbirth – and childcare – really can be as beautiful and natural as conception, if you have your babies in what we call the BabyLove way. This means that the arrival of a wanted child should bring a richer, more fulfilling relationship to the parents.

A BabyLove mum knows how important it is for every mother to stay a warm, responsive lover. Sensuous? Definitely! But not because she works non-stop at an array of erotic games. A BabyLove mother makes love not just with her body. She creates a world of love around her family. So she never needs to sort out her priorities. She would always rather be a champion cuddler than a first-rate cleaner. She'll put off the washing but reckons a peep-bo game won't wait. She knows that babies don't care if their clothes are hand-me-downs as long as there's a fresh supply of kisses every day. Simply put, she feels that loving mothering is more important than mothercraft. And because she has such a relaxed attitude to life and love, motherhood is never a wearying grind.

How often have you heard stories like this one from the mother of an eight-month-old boy: 'To me, being a mum means being tired all the time. I just want to sleep for a week. Even if Robert Redford walked into my bedroom, I'd say: "Don't take this personally, but I fancy a good night's sleep more. Wake me after that and then we'll see – maybe!" ' Believe us, a BabyLove mother would make time for Robert Redford!

But how can you live your life fully and be a mother at the same time? Simply carry the baby in a sling on your back and get on with living. And your baby will stay right where every baby loves to be – up close to mum. So you won't catch our kind of mother becoming a martyr to her child. And she's backed up by psychologists who say the more she sacrifices the more she'll resent her baby.

We believe that motherhood should not be all give and no get. In the same way that love-making involves enjoying yourself as well as pleasing your partner, your first priority should be to enjoy your baby. All you have to do is look at the world through your baby's eyes. Not because you're a slave to your child but because putting the baby's needs first means a more contented, less demanding child. And when you have a sweet-tempered little snugglepot to care for, motherhood isn't hard work, it becomes fun.

Too many mums miss out on any enjoyment right from the time they first become pregnant. A lot of women – and their fellas – still think that expectant mothers should only coddle themselves and think beautiful thoughts. Few people know that pregnancy can do wonders for their love life. (Find out *exactly* how it does – with illustrations – on page 65.)

Why shouldn't pregnancy be the most loving, tender, sexy time of your life? After all it's not as if you have to worry about birth control any more so making love can be more free and more fun. Remember, pregnancy isn't an illness and after the first few weeks you're probably feeling your energetic and beautiful best.

BabyLove mums know that although pregnancy is a serious time in a woman's life it can also be the most exciting. It doesn't have to mean an end to flirting, careers, parties or most sports. We know a dazzling lady whose divorce became final when she was 6 months pregnant. Her fit of the dooms soon blew away when she met a gorgeous Canadian 6-footer who said pregnant ladies turned him on. They had a crazy 10-day fling before he had to return home. We admired her not because she had an affair but because she *felt* like one! (And guess who became her second husband?)

Can pregnancy make you a sexier lady? American sex therapists Masters and Johnson say yes! Especially during the 5 middle months.[1] And Dr. Rosamond Bischoff, after 40 years as a London gynaecologist explains how it happens: 'The increased circulation of blood flowing to and from the womb during pregnancy produces extra pressure in the pelvic area and this increases a healthy woman's sex drive.

'Patients have come to see me complaining that they're itching or tingling and convinced there's something wrong. The 'something wrong' is that they're not making love often enough!'[2]

A BabyLove mum would never have that problem because she knows that a passionate love life can actually help her have an easier childbirth. Who says so? Dr. Sam Baxter of London's Charing Cross Hospital. He did a survey of sexuality and childbirth with a group of new mothers. Afterwards he told us: 'It struck me during this survey that the women who said they had orgasms in intercourse also had a much shorter labour.

'So you could say that orgasm is good practice for labour because the actions in the womb during both are practically the same.'[3]

Dr. Baxter thinks that childbirth is a psychosexual experience because the mind controls what the body feels. It works like this: society teaches women that childbirth equals pain. Therefore women expect pain. Therefore they feel pain. He reckons the opposite of all this may not be exactly true, 'but the right mental attitude can not only reduce pain a lot it can actually make having a baby a much more enjoyable experience.'

And Dr. Baxter has also found that one of the psychological factors linking sex and childbirth is a feeling of relaxation, or the ability to 'let go'. So far from limiting your love life pregnancy can actually enrich it. We've even heard of women who say they've had orgasms while actually giving birth, (though we've never met one). Sounds incredible? Not really. Dr. Bischoff says: 'Orgasms during delivery aren't as unusual as they sound. An orgasm is simply a state of ecstasy and different women experience that to different degrees.'

But what happens after the baby arrives and the hard work really begins? How can you be a mother and a lover when the baby has ruined your sleep three times in one night? And how do you make a man feel he's still the centre of your world when a baby takes up all your time? We had a lot of unexpected hassles when we first became mums. But they can be reduced to manageable size if you know what to expect and how to cope (which is what this book is all about). And especially if your man has been interested and involved in the baby from conception onwards. (*See* chapter 2.)

We believe dads should never be left out of the child-bearing and rearing business. Two people make a baby and ideally your child needs both for a loving, happy life. So although the welfare of the baby is important the relationship between the parents is just as vital. And when parents really go through childbirth *together* the arrival of a wanted baby is a link of love drawing them closer.

The switch from child-free couple to parents is the greatest change of life-style most people experience. Greater even than the change from singles to couple. And naturally, it involves a terrific adjustment. However, your new role as parents will depend largely on how strong your relationship is as lovers. This is the reason we feel a richly rewarding love life helps to ease a couple through the stresses of parent-hood.

So it's love that makes two people one. *Through* love they make a baby together. *With* love they share every aspect of parenthood. And when a couple truly share the responsibility of a child the work is halved but the love is doubled.

CHAPTER TWO

The Future Father

Three's company. But try telling that to some expectant fathers! They still think that babycare is just women's work. And when it comes to pinning a nappy on a wriggling bottom they reckon their large, manly hands just can't manage such a fiddly, small job.

Perhaps dads have always been content to watch from the sidelines because the experts have told them that's a father's role. Child psychologist John Bowlby's theories on motherhood relegated a generation of fathers to playing 'second fiddle'. His theory is 'by providing love and companionship they (fathers) support the mother emotionally and help her maintain that harmonious, contented mood in the atmosphere of which her infant thrives.[1]

We think this is not nearly good enough. A father shouldn't be an interested bystander. He should get right into the thick of the action! Where is it written that men get to spend hours drinking with their mates while women visit thrilling places like a clinic packed with colicky kids? Who said men get to watch all the new series on TV while women get to watch for the tell-tale signs of a reddened face and baby grunts that mean another nappy change? And what Voice from on High declared that only a female hand can rock a cradle?

Underlining this Dr. Fitzhugh Dodson, American psychologist, says: 'Fathers seem to be afraid of tiny babies and we don't know why. All we are sure of is that many fathers do stay away from young babies and that it is not good for the babies when that happens.'[2]

It usually seems to be much more difficult for a man to adjust to life with an extra small person in the home. But the rewards of fatherhood aren't earned without some effort. A baby can't love someone she doesn't know. Child psychologist Phyllis Hostler says that every father will 'if he is wise, share with the mother in the physical tending of the baby. For in this way, the child comes gradually to distinguish a second being whose stronger hands bath and change him occasionally and whose deeper voice soothes him.'[3]

So to a baby, a father has a definite role in her life, not just as a male 'mother'. There is always something one parent does better than the other. It may be persuading a reluctant feeder to eat. Or making the right kind of soothing noises at bedtime. Many fathers don't mind helping with the baby. But many working mums find that they are still left with most of the work.

Fathers who are shirking should listen to Phyllis Hostler. She adds: 'Actual physical care is the only expression of love that a baby can understand at first and through which she learns to love in return.'[4]

Building a Bond of Love

To build a loving bond between your man and your child you must first realise that masculine attitudes to babies and family life are very different from women's. Almost from birth little girls are given baby dolls and start learning to be mothers someday. But little boys not only never learn such lessons, they're actively discouraged from being so 'sissy'. From babyhood their interests are directed away from the family to the wider world outside. In their games they are action men – astronauts, paratroopers or Grand Prix racing drivers.

This conditioning is slowly starting to disappear but some men still resent the arrival of a baby because fatherhood may affect their free way of life. This attitude was summed up by the half-joking remark of a man whose second wife was having their first child, his third: 'Raising kids is your department. I don't know what to do with little babies. So just show him my photograph now and then for the first few years so he'll know who I am. I'll take over when he's big enough to try for the football team.'

Creating an atmosphere in which a man is willing to share the work as well as the fun of parenthood is the answer. And this should begin when you first tell him he's going to become a dad.

How to Tell Him

Too many women act as if they were going to have a virgin birth. They are so excited they forget that men made them mothers. So their attitude is: 'It's *my* body that's changing. *I'm* the one who gives birth. Therefore, it's *my* baby.'

This is the kind of thinking that can lead to a rift in any loving relationship right from the start. It doesn't acknowledge that a baby is the product of two people. From conception onwards you must be sure that your fella knows you are conscious of this. You both may have *suspected* it, but the way a man finds out he is *definitely* going to be a father, especially for the first time, is therefore crucial. The right moment can make all the difference, particularly if you're a little apprehensive about his reaction.

1 Don't tell him when he's tired or in a hurry like rushing off to work or the second he walks through the door home from work.

2 If he's a football fanatic it's no good bursting in on him half-way through 'Match of the Day'. You'll just have to wait for a time when you have his full attention.

3 Don't say: 'I'm pregnant' or 'I'm expecting a baby' or even 'You've made me pregnant'. From now on the word 'I' should be strictly limited in your vocabulary.

4 *Do* say something like: 'Something great has happened to us. *We* are going to have a baby.'

5 Or you could try a lighter approach like a colleague of

ours. One June morning she said to her bloke: 'What would you like for Father's Day?' He looked surprised: 'But I'm not a father.' She grinned: 'Yes, you are – I've just got my pregnancy report and it's positive.'

Father's Feelings

Don't be disappointed if your fella doesn't immediately leap up and down with excitement or start turning the spare room into a nursery. Many men take time to grow accustomed to the idea of fatherhood.

Letters to a national newspaper [5], on reactions from new fathers to be:

'The first words my husband said were: "Don't just stand there! Make me a cup of tea. I've had a shock".'
(From New Cross, London)

'The first time I told my husband he was going to be a father he hit the roof. And he was nearly in tears at the prospect that I would have to give up my good job. We are now divorced.'   (From Birkenhead, Merseyside)

'My husband's reaction was: "Damn! There goes my new Mini".'   (From Bradford, Yorks)

'After six months of marriage I was told I was pregnant. I rushed home, head in the clouds, expecting to be greeted with love and kisses. Instead, my husband shook my hand and just said: "Well done!" '
(From Whitefield, Manchester)

If your man has this kind of attitude, don't suspect he's allergic to children. It's just that apart from his upbringing he is also conditioned to think of himself as the family's financial lifeline – no matter how much his wife earns. So he may see the arrival of a baby in one way as a burden on the budget. Especially if you plan to give up work and become a full-time mum.

Even more important than money worries is the overriding fear that he will have to share your love with someone else. He suspects that a baby will take up all your attention and take you away from him. And who can blame him? No one enjoys being downgraded from star to supporting actor. It could lead to the sour comment that one now-divorced dad told a marriage guidance counsellor: 'I married a lovely sexy girl – then she turned into someone's mother.'[6]

We think you can still be the lovely sexy girl he fell for and a good mum but only with his help, so that both of you are caring for your baby. And both share the responsibilities, not only the mother. Asking too much? From some men, yes. If their conditioning goes too deep, they may simply feel that it's your job to care for the baby. If they think like that, they miss out a lot. But in spite of all the hassles, some fathers find they enjoy being dads *and* sharing the workload. Some famous fathers spoke to us about their feelings:

Paul McCartney:

'I talked to a lot of people before we had our first baby and a few said, you know older ladies said: "Don't go, it won't be pleasant. You won't like it." In the old days it wasn't the done thing to go and watch your baby coming. They said I'd only be in the way.

'Linda and I talked it over and she said to me: "Well what do you think?" And I said I'd like to be there. So we went along to a nursing home and they said, "You couldn't possibly stay here overnight." And I said "I've got to. I'm going to see the baby come". So I said "We'll have to go to another nursing home then – you know, a bit of bribery there." So they said they'd try and fix it up.

'Anyway, I had a camp bed beside Linda's bed. And when the time came for her to have the baby I was useless. She had to do it all. I was just terrible. But I got her to the clinic safely anyway. And I saw the baby, Mary, being born.

'For me, it was the most magic experience of my life because it was real and yet magic. It was real magic. And I thought: "How do they do that, it's very clever." We made love and suddenly all this happened.

'So anyway, I was there and I just tried to help Linda and comfort her. And say, you know "it's cool" and everything. And she had the baby and I was able to tell her it was a girl and say it's all over. And we both went back to her room, had a little bit of a chat and everything, so it was really nice because we could be really very intimate. She didn't have the experience on her own and then tell me about it. You know, I knew all about it with her. It was such a very close experience. We loved it. We like all that kind of closeness. If you're going to be married you might as well really be married. And kids are a big part of all that, very much – yeah!'[7]

Donald Sutherland:

'It was the most incredible, wonderful, terrifically joyful, sexual, sensual, loving time of our lives. It was so intensely personal that it's hard to believe we didn't discover it all by ourselves. But it is as common as dying or making love or being born. It's what the hospitals categorise as "normal childbirth" and it was extraordinary for us because we did it together.'[8]

Mick Jagger:

'I'm a fantastic dad! And Jade's a fantastic kid, a lovely baby, very sweet and good-tempered. Most babies seem to cry all the time but mine doesn't. Every time I look at her, she's just gurgling and smiling away to herself. I've always been a good father and this kid makes it easy to be that way.'[9]

Sylvester Stallone (Star of 'Rocky):

'My son, Sage, is a Taurus, a steadfast, loving sign. When my wife Sasha went into hospital I went with her. And the doctor said she won't have the baby for another 12 hours yet. I said "You're crazy – this kid has been planned to arrive at exactly the right conjunction of the stars. He'll be born within 45 minutes." Sage arrived 31 minutes later.

Watching your baby being born is fantastic – a miracle! Seeing all that makes you much more involved with your child. I think I'll make a lot more boys. If I had a daughter I'd be incredibly jealous. Do I change his nappies? Are you kidding? Of course I do. I call it the Dump Patrol. Whatever he dumps, we take turns to clean up. I believe in the family unit, being really involved with your kids. You don't get married or start a home if you don't feel that way.[10]

Alan Minter (European Middleweight Boxing Champion)*:*

'I think I'm a better fighter since I became a father. Being a dad has definitely helped me in my career. When I'm fighting, I think about my kid and I want to win for her although she's too little to know about it. I want her to know her dad was a champion and be proud of me. I'm crazy about my little girl. Even leaving her behind for a week while I had the title fight in Italy was hard. On the day of the fight, I got a card from my wife saying Kerry sends you a kiss. And it had her dribbles all over it. It really chokes ya. And it gave me that little extra boost for the fight.

'I wanted to see her born but there were a few medical problems so I couldn't. And when the doctor carried her out to show me, it was the only time I've really been knocked out.

'When my wife was pregnant, I used to worry because we always went out a lot. I thought a kid would keep us in. It's completely the opposite. We take our baby everywhere. And if we do stay in, she's the best show in town.'[11]

Ways to Involve Him

Try to help your baby's father to see what he's missing. This will mean some extra effort on your part. But remember it's not so much for your benefit or even his. It's for your baby's sake. No one is ever going to make him take an interest in the child if you don't. So here are a few ways to start a family romance.

1   When you are pregnant persuade a friend with a sweet-tempered baby to plonk her child suddenly into your man's arms. A friend of ours tried this ploy when she had to dash into the kitchen to rescue a burning dish. When she returned she found the expectant dad cooing at the child, and boasting to his lady: 'I'm really rather good with kids, you know.'

2   Suggest he goes with you to the father's night at your relaxation classes. This is a good way to make him understand exactly what's involved in childbirth. Once a man sees the enthusiasm and excitement of both the lecturer and other dads, he may be much more interested in the whole process of birth. That's the time to ask him if he will help you by being with you right through your labour.

3   When you bring the baby home from hospital and you give her a late-night feed, hand her over afterwards to her dad. No man could resist cuddling the warm, sweet-scented and contented little bundle snuggling into the curve of his neck.

4   Show him that you and the baby both really need him because it's easy for a man to feel excluded in your early days at home. Tell him you couldn't possibly manage without his help. Suggest he takes a turn with the dawn watch changing and feeding the baby at weekends to give you a break. (If you breast feed, you're usually on your own. Although one doctor we know tells the story of a very sleepy patient who was a new mum but who just couldn't wake up in the mornings. 'So her husband fetched the baby, changed him and arranged the baby on his mother's breast with pillows so that both mum and baby were comfortable. He read a good book or filed his nails till the baby was satisfied. Mum sometimes woke up, sometimes not. They all flourished.' Can we just add that he must have been a jewel of a husband!)

5   Babies love both skin contact and water play so put yours

in the bath with her dad. The fun they have together will do wonders for their relationship.

6 One of the newer ways to involve a dad in the birth of his child was started by Dr. William Hazlitt of Kingston, Pennsylvania. He not only allows dads to be present at the birth, he actively encourages them to deliver their own babies under strict medical supervision. Dr. Hazlitt says: 'I started this in 1967 when a father who had seen two previous deliveries asked if he could deliver his third child himself. It worked out very well as normal birth is a spontaneous process in which a baby slips out usually unaided. All a dad has to do is hold out his hands to catch his child.

'All parents tell me it's the most wonderful experience of their lives. And surprisingly the fathers are never nervous. A month before the due date I meet the father and give him a few tips. And he can review these with a nurse if he wants to. The only time I intervene in a delivery is if we take the baby's heart tones on a monitor and discover a problem. Only three or four per cent of births are Caesarean and only three or four per cent need forceps. So most births are natural, straightforward deliveries which can be handled by fathers.'

Compared with the time when a man stayed outside waiting to hear about the birth this is a much more satisfying way to involve himself in his baby right from the start.

CHAPTER THREE

Life Before Birth

Of all the millions of people in this world you and your man chose each other for the act of love which made your baby. In exactly the same way one single sperm out of the 400 million released by the man merges with one special, ripe egg. And that egg, fertilised with love, becomes your baby.

This beautiful union is astounding when you consider the odds against it happening. Your man's sperm have a tremendous upstream journey, swimming against body currents to reach the egg. The tadpole-like shape of the sperm helps in their struggle because the long tail propels them forward. This drops off when the head of one sperm penetrates an egg.

The journey of about 9 inches from the top of the vagina up through the womb and along the fallopian tubes takes about 45 minutes. The sperm have a lifespan of between 48 and 72 hours. So if no ripe egg meets one lucky sperm in the tubes during this time, all the effort is wasted.

While all this is happening inside your body you're probably in the relaxed slumber that follows love-making and are totally unaware of this miraculous process!

But just calculate the odds on one sperm reaching one egg and timing their meeting so that conception can take place. No wonder humans are called the most infertile beings on Earth. As one fertility expert told us: 'The world is over-populated, that's true. But if you think of the millions of copulations taking place every minute without any contraception you'll realise how few actually produce babies.'

Within a few hours after the sperm penetrates the egg it fuses with its nucleus to form one living cell. Soon, this cell begins dividing into two identical parts. Each in turn divides again. This process looks like a blossoming flower quivering as each new petal-like cell appears. This is called the embryo. In the next 280 days (the length of an average pregnancy) these cells continue to divide until a perfectly formed baby is ready to enter the world.

When the egg is fertilised and starting to divide, it makes its second most important journey – down the fallopian tube and into the womb. It floats along helped by waving hairs which coat the walls of the tube. After about seven days it reaches a comfortable position in the wall of the womb and beds down. Until the fertilised egg really establishes itself your pregnancy is still uncertain.

While all this is happening your body is busy preparing you to become a mum. First, the ovaries empty oestrogen into the bloodstream. This hormone acts on the lining of the womb so that it thickens. New blood vessels suddenly appear and your glands become more active. The reason for all this is to provide nourishment for the embryo.

Then the ovaries produce another hormone called progesterone. This fans the spark of human life in two ways. It soothes the womb by slowing down its normal contractions and helps the lining to secrete food for the new embryo. From this moment, until the time of birth, this egg will float securely in a bath of amniotic fluid. Two weeks after fertilisation the body is producing so much progesterone the menstrual cycle stops.

You are now beautifully pregnant and are just beginning to suspect it. But nervous ladies will still carry tampons in their handbags for weeks – just in case.

Points to Pregnancy

How do you know when you're pregnant? You'll first suspect when the date you've ringed on your calendar arrives and nothing happens. A missed period, if yours are normally regular, is one of the most reliable signs of pregnancy. Tingling, sensitive breasts and sometimes nausea are the other early warning signals.

You may also feel unusually tired or rush to the lavatory more often. (This is a result of the bladder becoming irritated by the pressure of the growing womb.) Sometimes, for no reason that doctors can explain, you *feel* totally different. It's almost like floating a few inches from the ground. This is why so many women are positive they're pregnant before having any tests.

Positive or Negative?

When you suspect you could be pregnant, make an appointment with your doctor. But don't be in too much of a rush. He may not be able to confirm your pregnancy until at least 14 days after your missed period was due. Your doctor will then arrange for you to have a pregnancy test at the pathology department of your local hospital.

Or, you could contact a local chemist who advertises quick pregnancy tests. These are about 98 per cent accurate but they'll put you out of your misery until you can see a doctor. (We know a girl whose pregnancy test was negative. But she went to her doctor anyway because she *felt* she was pregnant. She was right!)

Wherever you go for your test you should take a small sample of urine in a clean jar. One of us rushed to the chemist with a half-gallon jar in the fond belief that the bigger the sample the more certain the test's result. When asked 'Can you test this, please. I'm four days late', the chemist grinned and said: 'Come back in a fortnight. Then bring another gallon to be sure we've got enough.' And he handed over a regular specimen jar – it held about half an eggcupful.

Pregnancy tests can take just a few minutes. They are done with a simple chemical test. 12 days after your period should have appeared a hormone called chorionic gonadotrophin can be detected in a pregnant woman's urine. It shows up most strongly in the first urine of the day.

Guide to Your Inside

When you're pregnant you get used to physical check-ups at every ante-natal clinic. They're painless, last only a few minutes and after the first few you won't feel even the slightest embarrassment. To understand what the doctors say when examining you it's handy to know how your body is constructed. So here are the areas the doctor pays most attention to with their medical names and meanings:

Vulva: This is the general medical name for the entire external female genital area. (Don't confuse it with vagina.) In the vulva are four fleshy lips which protect the vaginal entrance. The two outer larger 'lips' are the labia majora. The two smaller inner ones are the labia minora. Where both sets of lips meet at the top is the clitoris.

Another part of the vulva is the entrance to the vagina and above it the urinary opening. Lower down is the anal canal.

Clitoris: This half-inch long, cylindrical-shaped tissue is the centre of a woman's sexual pleasure. It has no function except to increase sexual excitement.

Perineum: Another part of the vulva, this is a triangular area of skin between the bottom of the vaginal entrance and the front of the anal opening. During the delivery of a baby the perineum is stretched. To avoid any tearing of the skin an incision is usually made by the doctor to enlarge the opening and allow the baby's head through more easily. This cut is called an episiotomy. (More about this on p.140.)

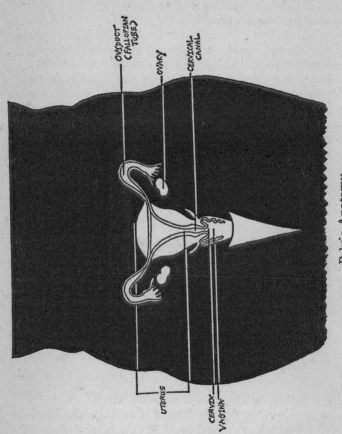

Pelvic Anatomy

Vagina: A tunnel about three or four inches long, its upper end is attached to the cervix which is the neck of the womb. Usually the vagina looks – as our friend, writer Claire Rayner describes it – like the collapsed sides of an empty toothpaste tube. But it is very roomy and elastic. When the baby's head comes through from the cervix this vaginal tunnel becomes the birth canal. And it stretches widely around the baby's head. (Remember, a baby's head is still disproportionately large for the body.) The vaginal tunnel is not only self-cleaning, it lubricates itself, too. And on either side of the entrance the Batholin's glands react to sexual excitement by swiftly increasing their supply of mucous. This secretion makes the vagina more receptive to sperm by neutralising the body acids which destroy them. So successful conception begins right here.

Uterus: A medical name for the womb. This is shaped like an upside-down pear, a hollow organ about three inches long. The baby lives and grows within it. And the womb enlarges with the size of the foetus.

Fallopian Tubes: They're like two little pipes, each curving outwards on either side of the womb. About four inches long and around a quarter of an inch thick they provide a route which the sperm follow from the womb to the ovaries. Fertilisation of an egg, the start of human life, takes place in the middle part of a fallopian tube.

Ovaries: Each woman has two ovaries which look like little olives in shape and size. They're on either side of the womb at the end of the fallopian tubes. Ovaries produce hormones as well as eggs.

Handling any Doubts

You're thrilled when your pregnancy is confirmed, of course. But soon after doubts may begin to creep in. One career girl we know had a typical reaction. She was horrified to find that in the middle of excitedly telling people her good news she was thinking: 'I don't even *like* small babies. And what's going to happen to our beautiful free life?' Other questions followed: 'Will we have to move to a larger house? Do I need to give up my job?' And she was really depressed to think that when it was too late she was really considering what parenthood meant for the first time.

A top London psychologist told us how common and very normal her feelings were. He said: 'This reaction is not unnatural even with women who have been trying to have a baby for years. Most have a fantasy of what it would be like to be a mum. As long as they aren't pregnant they can go on dreaming of sweet, smiling babies smelling of talcum powder who never need a nappy change. Just like those they see on television. As soon as they have conceived reality confronts them. So do the new responsibilities. Only then do they sit down and think about how a baby will actually affect their way of life. Usually this state lasts only a few days before it is overtaken by the happiness of the occasion. When the baby finally arrives most of them cope and they cope well.'

Nevertheless, you can't help worrying about the way a baby will change the lovely carefree life you and your man have been enjoying. Having a baby means seeing your favourite movie stars less often than the local health visitor. It means changing clothes with 'dry-clean only' tags for drip-dry bargains which can withstand little sticky fingers and puddle rings. It can even mean changing friendships – your second-best friend is no longer your hairdresser but your baby-sitter.

It involves always being prepared in a way only Boy Scouts bother about – like packing more nappies than you need just in case the car or train breaks down. And watching your baby's weight more carefully than your own.

If you dread the thought of such a drastic alteration to your lifestyle this doesn't mean that deep down you don't really want a baby. Dr. Dana Breen says that facing up to such feelings can help a woman 'towards a positive change, a greater understanding of herself'. And you should never bottle up these doubts, as Dr. Breen adds, it is 'probably healthier in the long run to express conflicts and fears'.[1] So talk out your worries with your man, your doctor or a close friend.

The Unborn Baby Grows

Studying the unborn child is a relatively new and uncharted field of research. But it may prove as thrilling as exploring outer space. With the latest techniques we can now peer into the inner space of the unborn. We can watch how they feel, hear, see – even dream.

Your baby is floating in a little space capsule (the amniotic sac) within your womb. And just like an astronaut the baby is tied to the mother ship's life support system by the umbilical cord. New Zealand scientist Dr. Margaret Liley gives us a peep into your unborn baby's world: 'An unborn baby is a water animal, a kind of combination between astronaut and underwater swimmer which lives in a water-filled balloon. The fluid in which it lives acts as a shock absorber and affords a constant temperature. If the mother falls or is pushed, it doesn't have much effect on it. Like an astronaut it enjoys the further advantage of weightlessness since the gravitational pull of the Earth has hardly any effect on it.'

The Development of Life Before Birth:

4 weeks: The spine, brain and heart are starting to form and a recognisable little creature is beginning to take shape.

6 weeks: Growing more human from nose to toes. The heart is beating. Buds of arms and legs appear. Very soon the face forms with eyes, eyelids and, at first, just a space for a mouth.

8 weeks: Halfway through the second month the embryo is just over half an inch (15 mm) long. By the end of this

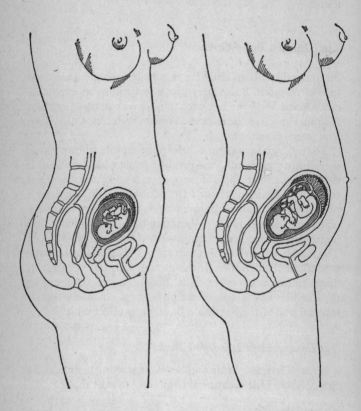

12th week   20th week

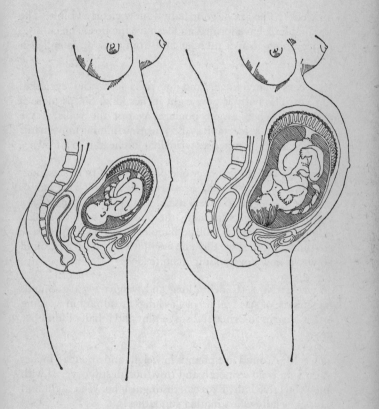

28th week   36th week

month the liver and stomach are developing. A small human can be recognised now though the head is disproportionately large.

12 weeks: The sex of your baby is now clearly visible. The vocal chords have formed and so have the lips. The embryo is beginning to flex muscles and from now on is called a foetus.

14 weeks: Tiny finger and toe nails form and eyelashes appear. The baby is now eight inches long. Sleeps most of the time. When awake bounces against the walls of the capsule, turns somersaults. Also makes swimming movements and occasionally practises wrinkling forehead into a frown.

24 weeks: Weighs just over one pound and is 12 inches long. The eyes are open and ears react to sound. The baby's personality begins to reveal itself. A budding rock 'n roll fan will bounce about and enjoy the pulsating throb of music. A more placid baby will be happier lulled to sleep by the rhythm of mother's walk. The first flutters you felt at around 20 weeks now develop into definite kicks.

28 weeks: Now 16 inches long and weighs 2-3 lbs. Stands fair chance of survival if born as lungs are almost in working order. Learns to drink and sips a pint and a half of fluid per day.

32 weeks: Around five pounds in weight and about 18 inches long. Skin is now smooth and rosy though still covered with fine protective hair. Eyes can distinguish between night and day, especially when mother sunbathes!

36 weeks: If a boy the testicles have now descended. A white protective waxy substance called vernix covers the skin. All limbs and organs perfectly formed, but resistance to germs still low.

40 weeks: Ready and willing to make a debut.

CHAPTER FOUR

First and Worst Weeks

A newly pregnant lady needs far more loving than she realises. Gynaecologist Rosamond Bischoff says: 'In the early weeks after her pregnancy is confirmed the more a woman makes love the more the baby will blossom and grow inside her.'

Dr. Bischoff believes intercourse does this by increasing the blood's circulation in the pelvic area: 'This makes the lining of the womb more juicy and soft. So the embryo snuggles down more deeply and the womb's walls hold it more securely.'

But often in these first tiring months love-making is the last thing on your mind. Conception starts some rapid internal changes in your body. One of these may transform your personality. A usually calm, even-tempered girl may burst into tears over an unimportant matter. Or flare up suddenly and begin a row. You may laugh crazily at something that never seemed funny before (and won't afterwards).

We know a girl who sat dry-eyed through Ali McGraw's death scene in *Love Story*. And scoffed: 'how ridiculous' when Vivien Leigh jumped off Waterloo Bridge. But when she became pregnant this hard-bitten movie fan got through three boxes of tissues when *Easter Parade* was re-run on television. Her husband walked in, looked at her and said: 'It's a happy musical, why are you crying?'

'I know,' she sniffed. 'But Judy Garland had such a sad life.'

People used to think the extra hormones flooding the system were responsible for the newly pregnant lady's strange moods. Certainly they play a part. But psychologists now believe that a woman's mental attitude may be an even greater influence on her personality. Psychotherapist Dana Breen warns: 'There is a danger in relying too heavily on a hormonal explanation of moods.'[1] She thinks this is a way for a woman of not facing up to her feelings and for the people around her to avoid their part in upsetting her.

And this happens when the people who treat a newly expectant mother don't allow her to take an active part in her pregnancy. So she ends up just submitting to the birth process. She may wait for hours at an ante-natal clinic then be whisked in and out without a chance to ask questions. Or, if she can snatch a chance to discuss her worries she finds they are scoffed at. And each time she visits the clinic she may see different doctors and never find out who they are. All of which makes her feel vulnerable at a crucial time in her life. Small wonder then that she gets upset easily.

Other Changes

The beautiful changes inside your body aren't often matched by what's happening outside. The effect of all those hormones surging through your system may be spotty skin, limp hair and lack of energy. So you could look pale, tired and sick. But console yourself that these first few weeks are the worst. Once you've survived them everything improves. (*See* chapter 6.)

The great plague of this stage is a terrible tiredness. You may feel totally exhausted all the time. Even a short walk from the bus to work seems a big effort. If you don't get a seat on the bus you almost feel like crying. But you don't look pregnant now so no one's likely to offer you one.

There are ways you can feel livelier. Don't try to cram too much into a day. It's better to sit quietly at lunch time rather than go window shopping with friends as you usually do. Try to use fewer bursts of energy. Do everything more calmly. Talk less. Walk more slowly. Work more steadily.

And avoid last minute panics.

Another nasty side effect of early pregnancy is nausea. Usually it's called morning sickness which is a crazy name because it can strike at any hour of the day. Recent research indicates that pregnancy sickness may be one more sign of a woman's inner conflict when adjusting to pregnancy. So it decreases as the pregnancy progresses and the woman gets used to her changed condition. Dana Breen adds: 'This explains why nausea and vomiting which are generally considered to be emotional reactions, occur with greatest frequency during the early months of pregnancy.'

Only one in every three pregnant women actually throws up. But many more feel queasy, especially early in the morning. If you feel really rotten it could be that you have a really strong baby. That's because the embryo while developing in the womb takes far more from your body than a less healthy baby. A really tough baby fights for nourishment and wins, but you may lose several meals.

Here's one way to minimise pregnancy sickness. Have a dry salty biscuit by your bed. When you open your eyes don't sit up. Just reach out and take the biscuit. Still lying down nibble and chew continuously until saliva starts flowing. (Avoid the old wives' remedy of the nice, strong morning cuppa. The tannic acid in tea will irritate an empty stomach so that you really throw up.) Anyway, it's common to loathe the taste of tea while pregnant.

Finally, sit up slowly. But when you do get out of bed don't sit down again for at least 20 minutes. This will ensure that the bile which has collected in your stomach can drain through to the intestines. Nausea only occurs when the stomach relaxes and lets bile rise.

No one need suffer the agonies of pregnancy sickness these days. You can get some perfectly safe pills from your doctor. But you must co-operate too by taking the stress off your body. To build a strong baby your system needs to concentrate all its energy on the pelvic area and your womb. So don't waste precious energy which could be used for your baby's benefit with unnecessary rushing about.

Ante-Natal Care

This is a series of regular checks on the health of you and your baby at free maternity clinics. Your initial visit to an ante-natal clinic is exciting because for the first time you're treated as a pregnant lady. Regular attendance at these clinics is essential for the well-being of both of you. Each visit is vital so it seems puzzling that a high proportion of expectant mums skip some weeks. Even if you feel well, that doesn't necessarily mean that all is well with the baby. For instance, toxaemia may not affect a mother's health noticeably at all, but her baby could be in grave danger. Only tests at the ante-natal clinic can alert her doctor to this problem.

You have three choices in ante-natal care. Clinics may be held either at your local maternity hospital or at your doctor's surgery. You can attend either, or split your treatment between them.

Your first visit, usually between the eighth and twelfth weeks of pregnancy, is the longest one. It starts with a lot of form-filling. You'll be asked for details about your past medical history, your family and their health, your menstrual cycle, and about any previous pregnancies.

You are weighed, measured, and your blood pressure is noted. This will be checked at every subsequent visit. Then the duty doctor will examine you in a private cubicle. He will give you a quick, general check-over then concentrate on your abdomen. Feeling the size of the womb with the flat of his hand gives him a guide to the baby's progress. Usually, he also carries out a gentle internal examination. You'll find this easier if you breathe out and relax your entire body. At many clinics this examination begins with a smear test which takes only a few seconds and is painless. A tiny amount of fluid is taken from the upper vagina for analysis. Occasionally this test shows up some cells with a tendency to become malignant.

Val: 'My smear test showed up some risky cells. The
doctors explained to me that this didn't mean I had

an early form of cancer, but simply a weakness in the cells which could turn cancerous – in three weeks, three months, thirty years or perhaps never.

'So in addition to my ante-natal classes I went to the gynaecology department of a hospital for regular examinations. The condition of the cells was closely watched, but, thank goodness, they didn't get worse. Three months after my baby was born I went into hospital again for a cone biopsy. This nicks out the affected cells and is completely pain-less. Since then I have had a total clearance at each check-up.'

After your smear test the doctor feels the size and position of your womb through the vagina. This is probably the last internal examination you'll have. After this, the growth of the womb can easily be gauged from the outside.

Urine tests:

The hospital usually provides you with a small, clean bottle for your regular sample of urine. You must bring this at each visit for testing. The analysts check it for protein which could indicate a kidney infection, or at a later stage, toxaemia.

Blood test:

This reveals your blood type and any signs of anaemia. It will also be checked for syphilis, which although rare, puts the baby at risk.

You will be asked to attend your clinic each month until you are about 28 weeks pregnant. After that you go fortnightly until the 36th week, and then weekly until admitted to hos-pital for the birth. You will be examined at each visit by the duty doctor, but at regular intervals, you'll probably be seen by a consultant gynaecologist. You may often have a long wait for examinations so take a book along (preferably this one!).

Ultrasound

Your doctor may ask you to take a special test if something is puzzling him. For example, one of our babies was much bigger than normal at one stage – or what is known as 'big for dates'. So the hospital arranged an ultrasound test. An ultrasound machine uses ultrasonic waves to trace a picture of the baby's shape in the womb on a screen.

Val: 'The doctor told me he wanted to screen my tummy to see if I was having one baby or two. I nearly fainted when I heard this because the idea of twins had never occurred to me. I was worried, too, about ultrasound. Would it hurt? I didn't know it then but it was one of the biggest thrills of my pregnancy.

'The ultrasound machine looks like an upside-down periscope attached to a unit full of knobs. In the centre is a miniature screen. You lie flat on your back on the table and olive oil is rubbed on to your tummy (the only part of you that needs to be nude. Discreetly draped towels cover the rest).

'Then the doctor moves the ultrasound "periscope" over your tummy, backwards and forwards, just touching it gently. This picks up the sound waves bouncing off the different parts of the baby's body in the womb. These sound waves are transmitted to the screen which forms a picture of the baby. Seeing that picture of my baby lying curled in my tummy was my most exciting moment. The doctor said he could not, at this stage, count the number of fingers or toes, or determine the baby's sex. But he could count babies and there was only one.'

Ultrasound is also used to spot severe deformities of the head or spine which occur in children with spina bifida. It can also show whether the baby's size is large enough for its stage of development. This would indicate that the baby was not being nourished properly by the mother's placenta. And ultrasound can reveal problems like placenta praevia in which the placenta lies below the baby blocking its exit from the womb. This usually means a Caesarian birth.

Amniocentesis

If you're 40 or over you may want a test to check that your unborn baby is normal. The chances of having a difficult or abnormal birth rise by more than 10 per cent after a woman is 40. This could mean having a Caesarean delivery or, even more serious, giving birth to a Mongol baby. (The medical name for this condition is Down's syndrome.)

To find out in advance whether your baby has Down's syndrome or suffers from spina bifida, you can have a test called Amniocentesis.

At 15 or 16 weeks the foetus begins to lose some of its cells in the amniotic fluid around it. Doctors can now draw out some of these cells with a needle inserted through the wall of the mother's abdomen. In most cases a culture can be grown from these cells which shows the chromosomes in each cell (and incidentally the baby's sex). If there is one chromosome too many the mother may have a child with Down's syndrome.

So it's vital to start your ante-natal care as early as possible in case it is necessary to arrange this test before the 16th week. But your doctor should warn you that there is a slight risk the test could endanger the pregnancy.

One of us was in hospital with Gill, an older mum who'd had a baby with Down's syndrome two years earlier. The baby had died after nine months' devoted nursing. When she became pregnant again she was naturally worried that this second baby might also be affected. So Gill had the amniocentesis test and waited a nail-biting month for the result. But as happens in 4 per cent of cases the test was unsuccessful and another was needed. When she had this second test she was 20 weeks pregnant and had another four weeks to wait before she knew the final result. Happily it proved negative. And when her beautiful, normal baby boy was born the whole ward celebrated with her.

Miscarriages

Miscarrying a baby may happen for one of three main reasons: something is wrong with the sperm or the egg; the embryo may not be securely planted in the womb, like a bulb which doesn't take root. Or there may be something wrong with what doctors call the maternal environment. For instance a woman may have an immature womb or she may consciously or unconsciously not want to have a baby.

A woman who miscarries her baby has feelings of grief, loss and depression even if she didn't want the child. But she can comfort herself with the thought that Nature has probably saved her from having a malformed baby. Almost a quarter of pregnancies end in miscarriage usually within the first eight weeks. Many happen so early that a woman hasn't even realised she was pregnant. But miscarriages can also occur much later in pregnancy. And some doctors believe the thalidomide drug produced deformed babies because it may have tranquillised wombs so much they were unable to throw out the damaged eggs.

If something does go wrong you'll get a warning sign – probably a loss of blood. If this happens tell your doctor immediately. If you have a history of miscarriages your doctor may be able to do something at an early stage to prevent the pregnancy aborting. But in general we believe you shouldn't try to stop Nature doing its work. So don't coddle yourself in the decisive early weeks of pregnancy. Don't go to bed early every night unless you're tired. And don't spend all your time sitting around with your feet up.

Instead, go about your life as normally as possible.

Doctors think there is only one time to protect a newly fertilised egg. And that's when your third period would have been due. Around that time, when the placenta is forming, you should have relatively early nights and a less hectic social life for about a week.

Miscarriages cannot be caused by sudden shocks, falls or strenuous exercise. An American obstetrician, the late Alan Guttmacher once said: 'You cannot shake a good human egg loose any more than you can shake a good, unripe apple from the tree. If you could there would be no more work for abortionists.'[2]

After a miscarriage some doctors used to advise waiting for three months before trying again. But new thinking is that a couple should start a family again as soon as possible. This is because hormone levels are high in the woman's body and this helps her to conceive. Mostly, miscarriages are simply bad luck. All the experts agree that nine out of ten young women who miscarry in their first pregnancy will deliver a healthy baby next time.

Who Will Your Baby Look Like?

Every baby is an equal mixture of both its parents. And every parent can't help wondering if the baby will have dad's big snozzle or mum's little turned-up nose. One small mum married to an extremely tall man spent her whole pregnancy with a mental picture of a baby with her short dumpy legs and its dad's long dangly arms, a little monkey brushing the ground with its hands as it walked.

Of course, Nature makes sure that babies' limbs and features are generally arranged in the right proportions. But whether your baby will wear glasses just like you, be musical like your sister, or go bald early like grandad depends on the body cells of the parents. Each cell in the baby's body is made up of 46 minute substances called chromosomes, 23 from the father and 23 from the mother. Each chromosome comprises tiny chemicals which contain the blueprint of your baby's looks, build and personality.

These genes in chromosomes control the way your child grows and develops, not only in the womb, but right through life into old age. One of these inherited traits is eye colour. If you and the father both have brown eyes your children should also have dark eyes. But if you have a relative with light coloured eyes there is a slight chance that one of your children could have blue or green eyes too. In the same way dark-haired people are more likely to have children with brown or black hair. Generally, dark genes are more powerful than light ones so they're called the dominant genes.

Skin genes are the exception to this rule. When a dark-complexioned parent marries a light skinned mate their children usually have medium toned skin.

But there is no guarantee that just because you and your husband are lively, out-going extroverts that your children will be the same. When it comes to looks and personality the law of averages is on your side, but Nature still springs some surprises.

How intelligent your child will be is quite a different matter. Experts cannot agree whether heredity is more important than environment. Generally, bright parents have bright children, but whether this is because intelligent people encourage their children to learn or whether the children were born smarter than average has never been satisfactorily proved.

Everything about your baby from the way she wrinkles her nose to the shape of her toenails comes half from you and half from your man. So she will resemble you both in some way. But the combination of her parents' genes will also produce a unique person.

Will My Baby be Normal?

Underneath the happy excitement of every pregnant mother lurks the fear that her baby will be imperfect. Her anxiety grows if there is some health problem in her family such as an aunt with a nervous disorder or a cousin with a cleft palate. She may even worry over something quite minor like flat feet or clumsiness.

Most babies are born perfectly normal and only between a tiny three and five per cent have any imperfections. These are mostly not serious – like a hare lip. So the chances of giving birth to a severely handicapped child are very small. However if there is any inherited illness in your family such as haemophilia or diabetes you will be asked about it at your first ante-natal clinic visit. But because your mother and grandmother had diabetes it does not necessarily mean your baby will also suffer from such a defect.

Home Delivery

The time to start planning to have your baby at home is in the first three months. For full information on organising a home delivery write to: The Society to Support Home Confinements, 17 Laburnam Avenue, Durham.

Mrs. Mary Whyte who heads the society says: 'It is easier to arrange home confinements if you live in a big city. But it may be very difficult in rural parts of Britain, especially in these English counties: Hampshire, Middlesex, Surrey, Bedford, Buckinghamshire, Gloucestershire, Merseyside, Devon, Cornwall, North Tyneside, Northumberland, West Sussex, parts of Sheffield, Yorkshire, and most of Scotland and Wales.' Where cuts in public spending have reduced the home birth service, you may have no choice at all.

You can find out about home births from your Area Nursing Officer. Get the address of yours from your local town hall or library.

Mrs. Whyte adds that it is your legal right to have your baby at home if you wish. But doctors don't advise home confinements if you are having your first child, your fourth or more, if you are under 20 or over 35, if you are less than five feet tall, and if you've already had a miscarriage or a medical complication like heart disease.

A good compromise may be the Domino system which has been operating successfully in some parts of South-East England. A midwife goes into hospital with the mother, delivers the baby, and about six hours later takes them home and is responsible for their care.

Tips for a Newly Pregnant Mum

If your pregnancy has just been confirmed what can you do right now to give your baby the best start to life? Here are four important points to remember.

1   Make love as often as you want to. This won't hurt your baby. On the contrary, as we've shown, frequent love-making will help your pregnancy to blossom beautifully.

2   Start practising for an easy birth now by strengthening the muscles of your vagina. Learn the pelvic floor exercise (*see* Slinky Sexercises, page 216). This easy training for labour can also improve your sex life, so it's never too soon to start this one!

3   Start protecting your unborn baby now! By giving up smoking (and riding in smoking carriages on trains, sitting in smoky cinemas). And ban all stodgy, starchy, sweet and sticky foods that don't help to build beautiful babies.

4   And while you're concentrating on all of the above as well as the marvellous changes within your body, try not to let it show too much. Don't be so self-absorbed that you push into the background the man who made you a mother.

CHAPTER FIVE

Do's, Don'ts and Definitely Nots

Every mother wants her baby to arrive in perfect condition. And the fact that so many babies do is almost miraculous because the nine months before birth are the most important and hazardous in the life of your child.

So you should give as much attention to your baby's welfare *before* birth as afterwards. It has been found that only a minute percentage of births, about 2 per cent, have any serious abnormalities and 80 per cent of these have no hereditary basis. So most of these defects might be avoided.

A few are the result of Nature's mistakes so you can't blame yourself for them. But many defects are man-made and you can prevent these though this may mean altering the habits of a lifetime. Like giving up smoking or changing your diet completely.

But any sensible, caring mother will want to do everything in her power to give her baby the best possible start to life. To guide you through the 40 weeks of normal pregnancy here are a dozen Do's, seven Don'ts, and a long list of Definitely Nots. Some may be easier to follow than others. But all are important if you want to avoid bearing a child who may be badly affected by the way you live.

Do's

1 DO think of your pregnancy as a natural state and not an illness. So live life as normally as possible.

2 DO make love as often as you feel like it right throughout your pregnancy. Intercourse actually aids your baby's development. (*See* chapter 6.)

3 DO attend every ante-natal clinic. Feeling well is no excuse for missing one of these regular health checks. The one you miss may be the one that could have saved your baby some distress.

4 DO have a rest daily – even if it's just sitting with your feet up while you go on working. This will keep you more active longer each day.

5 DO see that you eat a balanced diet. Being well fed isn't the same as being well-nourished. For example a hamburger and chips will give you some protein but a lot more calories. If you substitute a fresh mixed salad for the starchy chips and the hamburger bun, you'll have a much more nourishing meal. (*See* Diet and Health, page 58).

6 DO have other topics to talk about besides babies. Your pregnancy may be a fascinating and unique experience to you. But it's just another ordinary birth so far as your friends are concerned.

7 DO keep up your usual amount of exercise. Don't sink into a chair every chance you get. But also don't go on five mile hikes before breakfast. Aim for the happy medium to have a happy pregnancy.

8 DO act on any advice the doctors at the ante-natal clinic give you. If they think you should do something like eating more or less, do it! Too many women promise doctors to do as they suggest then do only what suits them. Your doctors have good reasons for their recommendations. If these are not clear ask for an explanation.

9 DO be sensible about long, unnecessary journeys. Now is not the time to tour the stately homes of Britain.

10 DO go to your doctor immediately if any of the following danger signs appears: unusual swelling of the face, ankles and feet or hands and fingers; any pain in the abdominal area; continuous headache and blurring of vision; a rush of water from the vagina or any bleeding. If you have a really bad fall see him at once. Don't worry about the baby – she is better protected than you think. (*See* page 61).

11 DO check that your underwear isn't too tight, especially bras. Choose knickers which don't have elastic that's too tight.

12 DO stay in charge of your own pregnancy. At every stage ask questions and make the major decisions yourself. If you are worried about anything at any time, speak up. An interested, aware mother gets better attention. And do make sure you find out about maternity benefits, and family allowances. (*See* chapter 21.)

Don'ts

1 DON'T stop working too soon unless your doctor advises it. Being away from your regular life and friends can be very depressing at the end of a pregnancy and may make the waiting seem endless.

2 DON'T move house during your pregnancy.

   Judy: 'We decided to move from a small flat and buy a a house when I became pregnant. As time was running out we didn't have many months to look around for the right place for us. So we got desperate and bought the first one that seemed suitable. I spent the last weeks of my pregnancy in a flap organising painters, carpet fitters and making curtains. It was the biggest mistake of our lives because we didn't like the house or the furnishings we bought in such a rush. Worst of all, my husband had to do all the packing himself and organise the move without me. The job became more difficult when the removal firm we hired turned out to be pioneers in sex equality. They sent one slightly-built girl to do the removal. So the whole job literally fell on to his shoulders.'

3 DON'T throw the home you've got into total upheaval to make room for the expected baby. That small person will take up a tiny amount of space. So fit the baby into your home. Don't fit the home around the baby. Wait until the baby is a few months old before finally deciding how to rearrange the furnishings.

4 DON'T compare pregnancy notes with friends. Each expectant mother is different and may need different treatment.

5 DON'T use the traditional pregnancy food cravings as an excuse to over-eat. Telling people you can't live without wine gums or cheesecake may fool them – but not your bathroom scales.

6 DON'T be constipated. There's no need for this if your diet contains the necessary roughage like fresh fruit and vegetables, muesli, bran and wholewheat bread.

7 DON'T put on much more than 28 pounds during your pregnancy. An overweight mum is far more likely to have a difficult birth and other complications. (*See* page 62.)

Definitely Nots

1 NEVER smoke during the whole 40 weeks of your pregnancy (and afterwards, if you can). Women who do smoke, have twice the miscarriage rate, almost a third

more still-born babies and over a quarter more babies die soon after birth. Smokers' babies are smaller at birth and in later life, are more likely to suffer with respiratory troubles. At school age, they'll still be smaller than their friends and may also have learning difficulties. This is because smoking reduces the amount of oxygen supplied to the baby in the womb. Smoking by the mother also affects the baby's blood supply. The British Perinatal Mortality Survey found that 1,500 more babies would survive every year if their mothers did not smoke. Ask your man to help by giving up cigarettes too.

2   NEVER drink heavily during pregnancy. Alcohol has now been linked with malformed babies and also with retarded mental development in babies whose mothers regularly drink to excess.

3   NEVER use a douche during pregnancy (or at any other time). A douche, which forces water into the vagina as recommended by some old wives tales, if you develop an itch is not advisable. Don't try and treat yourself. Report it to your doctor at your next ante-natal clinic (or before, if it's worrying you). The forced douche can make infections worse rather than cure them.

4   NEVER have an X-ray *ever* except in the 10 days following a period in case you're unknowingly pregnant and that includes dental X-rays. X-rays are particularly dangerous for expectant mums and could lead to forms of cancer such as leukemia in the baby. Large doses of radiation could kill an unborn child.

5   NEVER fail to tell the doctor immediately if you come into contact with any infectious disease like German measles.

6   NEVER vary from the course the doctor sets you if you suffer from diabetes. It is vital for the survival of your baby to maintain exact blood sugar levels.

7   NEVER lose your cool if you can possibly help it. Stress raises the blood pressure during pregnancy and may lead to toxaemia which literally starves your baby of oxygen in the womb. A mother-to-be who is going through a bad time in her marriage or any traumatic experience will need more rest than usual, although doctors note that unmarried mums who must be subject to higher than average stress, usually produce perfectly normal babies. But pregnancy puts an enormous strain on your body so don't add to this by overworking unnecessarily. And don't become anxious about any aspect of your pregnancy. This is why we think you should ask as many questions as you want so that you understand what's happening to your body – and the baby – at all times.

8   NEVER over-extend your energy if you suffer from high blood pressure. This is called hypertension. But you can reduce its dangerous effects on your baby by sticking to a salt-free diet. Also get plenty of rest and relaxation. Give up smoking and drinking and never miss a single ante-natal clinic. Watch your weight, too. In this, as in all other potential dangers, you may feel fine. But your baby may be sending out distress signals which only regular health checks will pick up.

9   NEVER, NEVER take drugs of any kind during pregnancy unless specifically prescribed by your *own* doctor. And that means ordinary, everyday family friends like aspirin. Even if a doctor prescribes a drug, be wary of taking it. Remember if you haven't a bulge, he may forget you're pregnant, especially if he's in a group practice and not your regular physician. Some doctors, aware of this risk, put a bright red star on the record card of any pregnant patient.

Judy: 'I get hay fever in summer and when I was a couple of months pregnant, I got my usual anti-histamine pill prescription from the doctor. I took the prescription to my regular small chemist shop near the office. He had done my pregnancy test so he knew. And he said: "It's probably perfectly harmless but drugs are never a good idea during pregnancy. Do you really want to run the slightest risk of harming your baby?" I used nose drops instead of pills that summer.'

It's best to keep off everything and anything, even pills and potions you've relied on for years like sleeping pills, tranquillisers, cough mixtures or headache cures. For example, regularly taking headache powder or tablets containing aspirin, phenacetin, codeine or paracetymol may damage a developing baby in various ways. These could range from anaemia in the newborn while the mother could tend to lose more blood and have a longer labour.

Okay, so does it really matter if you take an aspirin or some other painkiller while pregnant? Yes, it does. Recent research shows that some people may be more vulnerable than others when it comes to drugs. A slight impairment of their body's make-up puts them just below the danger threshold. So when they take a drug it may have more effect on their body and the baby they are carrying, than on dozens of people. The trouble is, there is no way yet known to detect the mothers at risk from everybody else. The only way to be sure, is not to take anything your own doctor does not prescribe.

If you think we're being scarey, remember in an adult most unexpected side-effects of drugs can be treated. But their effect on an unborn baby is irreversible and can lead to abnormalities. One expert sums up the risk to babies before birth in this forceful way: 'The months before birth are the most eventful part of life and we spend them at a rapid pace. At the beginning the body consists of one cell; by the time of birth, it has two hundred billion cells.

'We do know from tragic experiences of recent years that the embryo is more sensitive to harmful actions of the environment than at any other period of life.'[1]

A survey in Scotland showed that during pregnancy, over 97 per cent of 1,369 women took medically prescribed drugs and 65 per cent took self-prescribed drugs. Significantly more of the mothers who took drugs had malformed babies. So if you're ever tempted to take some remedy without checking with your doctor first, bear in mind this terrible fact: most malformations in the newborn are the result of outside influences on the mother, almost always preventable.

To sum up: avoid everything that contains drugs of every type unless your doctor – aware of your condition – prescribes them. Even your regular anti-flu jab. And that goes not only for pregnant women but those who are hoping to be! Would-be mums should also be aware of another heartbreak hazard. If they forget to take a contraceptive pill, and, becoming pregnant unknowingly, then continue with the pill, their babies stand a chance of being born with heart defects. This is the finding of a 7-year study in America on over 50,000 expectant mothers. The moral of the story is never, ever forget to take your pill.[2]

Eating for a Healthy Baby

The loveliest ladies-in-waiting know that the secret of building a beautiful, healthy baby lies right in front of you, on your dinner plate. Not only are you what *you* eat, but your baby is, too. A baby can't develop healthily if her mother is living on junk food like chips, baked beans, cakes and biscuits.

But this doesn't mean you have to live through a boring nine months of weight watching and calorie counting. It's simply a matter of choosing to eat foods which promote health and not those which damage it. And with a dash of imagination, your taste buds will appreciate the change, too. For example, say you normally lunch on pork sausages with instant mashed potatoes, frozen peas and bread and jam, and cream cakes with your afternoon tea. A better – and just as filling – meal for a mum-to-be is roast chicken with fresh greens, jacket potatoes, steamed carrots with a wholewheat brown roll. Instead of cream cakes, have a fresh orange or apple. Both meals may be delicious. But the second, more healthy one is higher in protein, lower in starch and the food is closer to its natural state because it is fresh.

During pregnancy, it's a good idea to avoid whenever possible all processed, packeted, tinned or preserved foods which all contain chemicals and additives. Refined foods lack roughage, necessary to prevent one of the hazards of pregnancy, constipation. So choose fresh fruit salad instead of frozen mousse. A piece of fresh cheese will do your baby more good than a mid-morning sticky bun, however much you crave it. The fresher your food, the more vitamins it contains. Every expectant mum needs a diet of bone-building, tissue-enriching protein and infection-fighting vitamins to build a beautiful baby.

This healthy diet really pays off. The famous American nutritionist Adelle Davis has shown that babies are born stronger and their mothers' labour is easier when their diets are well balanced.[3] There is also strong evidence that if women eat well, they have stronger, more alert babies. During World War II, pregnant mums got priority in food rations in Britain. Even though the food available was very limited, the stillbirth rate dropped by 25 per cent. It's a fact that the British people were never more healthy during wartime when starchy, sugary foods like sweets were not available.

Another bonus of good nutrition during pregnancy has an almost instant effect. Cutting out fatty fried foods reduces nausea which is often aggravated by the smell of greasy food frying. It also means fewer spots, too!

If you eat wisely, you'll banish the twin terrors of every pregnant woman: tiredness and irritability. To do that, you need to eat lots of foods rich in B vitamins like whole meal bread, spinach, wheatgerm, from chemists (Bemax) and liver (smother it in onions if you dislike liver. Or grill it with bacon and herbs. Or combine with yoghurt sauce or an orange sauce.)

A good diet for a day in the life of an expectant mum could be: two eggs poached on wholemeal toast with a glass of orange juice (preferably freshly squeezed). And a large glass of a special milk cocktail to help you have a peppy pregnancy. Make the cocktail like this: fresh, cold milk with two tablespoons of dried skimmed milk powder for extra protein, whisked in. Add a little brewer's yeast (buy it from the chemist) plus a dash of vanilla or a fresh banana if you wish. This high protein drink with the breakfast will help you boost your blood sugar level right through the day so you shouldn't feel hungry or tired, even if you lunch late.

For a mid-morning break, have an apple, piece of cheese and crispbread if you need it. Have a cuppa if you fancy it. At lunch, choose a sardine or chicken salad or a mackerel with fresh green vegetables (or salad). And for supper, a serving of liver or lean beef or lamb or pork with fresh vegetables, wholemeal bread and fresh fruit salad or yoghurt to follow. Another milk cocktail before bed will bring your milk intake up to at least a pint every day which is your minimum.

Why are these foods so important? The right combination during your pregnancy contains all the proteins, vitamins and minerals which are essential – not only to you but to your growing baby.

Here's what each does for your body and your baby:

Protein: Helps the building of tissue, a good, solid placenta and a strong womb. Keeps the blood sugar (which governs how energetic you feel) at a consistently high level. Foods containing protein: meat, fish, eggs, cheese, milk, beans.

Vitamin A: Helps resistance to infection and has an effect on your eyesight. Foods: fresh vegetables, milk, skimmed milk (and remember, fresh vegetables are great laxatives).

Vitamin B: Thought to prevent nervousness, skin complaints, bowel problems and fatigue. Foods: wholemeal bread, liver, brewer's yeast, wheatgerm (Bemax).

Vitamin C: Counteracts the effects of eating junk food,

bacteria and viruses in your body. Keeps cell walls strong and also helps to get the placenta strong. Good at helping the body to absorb iron. Foods: lemons, oranges and grapefruit.

Vitamin D: With calcium, strengthens bones and tissues and helps the body to use calcium in blood to strengthen tissue and bone cells. Foods: mackerel, sardines or any oily fish, sunshine (use sunray lamp if you have one, strictly according to instructions).

Vitamin E: Helps heating processes. Governs amount of oxygen you use, helps to process foods strong in Vitamin A. Foods: sweetcorn, corn on the cob, peanuts, eggs, wholemeal bread.

Folic Acid: Helps to guard against anaemia and tiredness Important to have daily doses as the body cannot store this Crucial for the formation of blood and new body cells. Foods leafy green vegetables like spinach.

Iron: Main ingredient of good, healthy blood supply and prevents anaemia. Helps carry oxygen to the baby and your cells. The baby also stores some of your own iron in her liver to draw on while living on a diet of milk only. As women rarely have enough iron, you'll need a supplement of iron tablets (from your ante-natal clinic). Foods: liver, egg yolks, fish, raisins and leafy green vegetables.

In the last two months before your baby is born, it's important to step up your intake of some important foods because this is the time when the brain is developing at a fast rate. So increase foods containing vegetable oils like olive oil, soya bean oil, peanut butter, avocado pear and wheat-germ (Bemax). Eat the oils as salad dressing or for cooking. Keep them in a fridge to stop them going rancid.

10 Questions every Expectant Mum Asks

Q. *If I accidentally fall, will this harm my baby?*
A: Many women have fallen flat on their faces without

hurting their babies in any way. This is because the fluid in the womb in which the baby floats, acts as a shock absorber. And the soft walls of the womb bounce away from any impact.

Q: *Why have I got a funny brown line running from my navel down into my pubic hair?*

A: The medical name for this is the Linea Nigra and it may appear around the 14th week of your pregnancy. No one knows why. It is caused by a darker pigmentation of your skin. You can't bleach or wash it away. It's more noticeable if you're a brunette but if you're redheaded, you may not have one at all. Soon after the birth, this line begins to fade though it may be several months before it vanishes completely.

Q: *If I put on a lot of weight during pregnancy, will my baby be bigger?*

A: Yes, according to Dr. Gordon Bourne, consultant obstetrician and gynaecologist at St. Bartholomew's Hospital, London. Mums who put on excess weight during their pregnancy tend to have heavier babies than those women who have watched their weight. But remember that if you do put on too much weight, you have a higher risk of developing complications like toxaemia which may endanger the baby.[4]

Q: *Will a maternity girdle make me more comfortable towards the end of my pregnancy?*

A: No. And it won't be good for your figure after the birth either. A girdle makes stomach muscles lazy by helping to do their job. Good posture is far better for your baby – and your figure – than any girdle.

Q: *Are there any sports I should avoid during pregnancy?*

A: It all depends on what you've been used to doing. If, all your life, you've been riding horses, then you can keep on riding – as long as your doctor doesn't ban it.

But if you've never been in the saddle nor played active sports regularly, don't start now.

Q: *Does every pregnant woman get stretch marks?*
A: No. It really depends on how much weight the mother gains and how elastic her skin is. Stretch marks are caused by the elastic fibres of the skin becoming over-taut. The original reddish marks fade to a silvery colour over the years but may never completely disappear. Many women believe that oiling your body with olive or baby oil will prevent these marks on abdomen and breasts. Doctors don't always agree but say it does no harm.

Q: *Will the baby be harmed if I sunbathe?*
A: No. Suntanning *in moderation* can be good for expectant mums because the action of the sun on your skin produces Vitamin D which is great for building your baby's bones.

Q: *How soon after the birth can I begin to use tampons again?*
A: Physically, you're ready after your post-natal check-up, unless your doctor advises against using internal sanitary protection. But many women find it more comfortable to use sanitary towels for a few months after birth.

Q: *When will my periods start again?*
A: If you're breast feeding, you won't have a normal period until you wean. But be careful – you can conceive while breastfeeding so see your doctor about contraception. If bottlefeeding, the menstrual flow may start about 28 days after the baby's birth. But some women are lucky and don't start for several months after the birth. The first period is usually longer and heavier than usual.

Q: *How soon can I carry heavy shopping after the birth?*
A: Not for at least eight weeks afterwards. A new mum

may not go shopping – but don't forget that full nappy buckets are often heavier than a week's shopping. So is a baby bath full of water. Don't lift any heavy object until your stomach muscles and womb have settled back to normal, around 8 weeks.

CHAPTER SIX

How To Be a Mother and a Lover

When lovers change into parents what happens to their loving? Many couples find that love-making during this time can be more magical, more erotic and even more fulfilling. So pregnancy does not have to mean the end of a satisfying sex life as many people still think. The changes in a woman's body make her more sensitive to her man's touch. And call for a more tender response from him. His new gentleness and concern makes her feel more loved – and therefore more loving in return. As any psychologist will tell you when a couple have a good, physical relationship, a normal, healthy pregnancy can make it even better. The ever-growing bulge between them is visible proof of their joy in each other.

Maintaining a happy sex life particularly at this time is vital for the future of your partnership. As Dr. Kjell Nilsen, a Scandinavian obstetrician now working in Britain, father of two young children, says: 'One third of all divorces occur in the first four years of marriage – that is, when children are starting to arrive. It seems obvious therefore that there must be a link between pregnancy and the start of marriage breakdowns.'[1] And when sex therapists Masters and Johnson studied the effect of pregnancy they found that many men first break their marriage vows when their wives are pregnant and intercourse has stopped.[2]

But pregnancy need not change a happy relationship says gynaecologist Rosamond Bischoff: 'Pregnancy can *improve* a relationship instead of wrecking it. It all depends whether the couple can adjust happily to the changes pregnancy brings.

'After all, the arrival of a baby means you're no longer just a couple, you're a family,' Dr. Bischoff explains. 'Do you want your man to be contented or frustrated as you go through this big change together? Love-making will make all the difference. Of course, this will mean changing the way you normally make love. For instance, temporarily giving up the so-called missionary position with the man on top. This doesn't mean your love-making is limited. Just the opposite! Finding newer, more comfortable ways to make love can be a lot of fun, and add spice to your love life, too.'

So sometimes people get lovely surprises. As this Hertford-shire mother and her husband discovered: 'I've got to admit that my bloke was never a great lover. Maybe because neither of us had much experience before we got married. But boy, did that change once I was pregnant! Every month I seemed to feel more sexy. Perhaps I lost a lot of hang-ups about my body with all those examinations at the clinic. Anyway, whatever the reason, my old man really responded to his hot new lady. He even went out to buy some sex manuals. And I started going to bed nude for the first time in my life. Thinking back on it now makes me wonder if we could afford another baby soon.'

Some women are surprised to find their sex drives get stronger right through pregnancy. But Masters and Johnson found the majority enjoy love-making most in the middle five months. 82 per cent reported much more excitement in their sex lives – better than anything they'd known before.[2]

Love in the Round

Set out below are six positions generally recommended for making love with a baby bump between you. These are not the only safe ways to have intercourse. But we hope they'll inspire you to discover some fun variations of your own. Remember, it's not what you do it's the way that you do it!

Tenderness turns a woman on far more than any advanced techniques – and this is especially true when she is pregnant.

Lightly brushing the insides of her thigh with the fingertips is far more arousing than wild clutches and heavy-handed grabbing. As a leading sexologist, Dr. Alex Comfort forcefully reminds us: 'Male strength is a turn-on in sex, but it isn't expressed in clumsy hand work, bear-hugs and brute force.' And he adds: 'Few people want to be in bed on any terms with a person who isn't basically tender and most people are delighted to be in bed with the right person who is.'[3]

So, to enjoy yourself in bed gently do whatever comes naturally to you both. After all, you know best what you like. Don't try too hard to do so-called sexy things – thinking all the time, 'Now I must kiss him here', or, 'Tickle him there', and then apply Part A to Part B.

Just as when you're not pregnant success in love-making comes from a loving awareness of what your partner is feeling. And this is shown in the way you touch each other. And don't try to hurry your pleasure. Anyone can grind out a tune on a violin. But it takes time and loving dedication to play really fine music.

No 1 Spoon style: The woman lies on her side. The man on his side behind her. Their bodies lie as close as two spoons in a cutlery drawer. Although not face-to-face this position leaves the man's hands free to caress her body. (If you're over 8 months pregnant, place a pillow under your tummy for more comfort.)

No 2 Face to face: The couple lie on their sides facing each other. She places her top leg over his. The man rests his top leg over her bottom one. As the baby bulge grows both partners should move their top halves further apart until they form a 'V' shape on the bed.

No 3 Double-decker: The man lies on his back. The woman lies face up on top on him. This position is most comfortable in the early months before the woman becomes large and

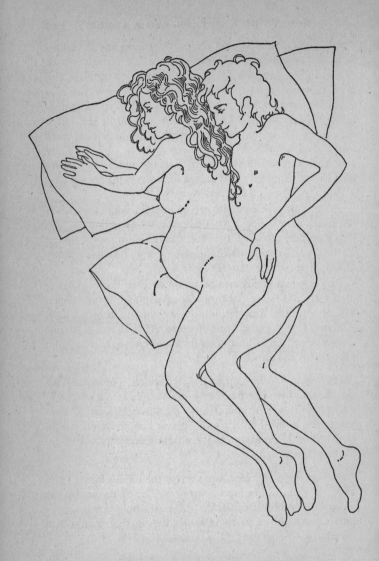

Spoon Style

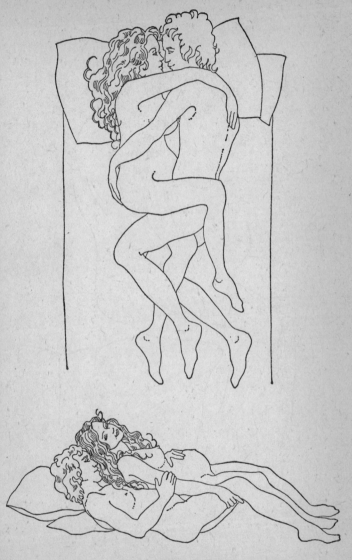

Above: Face to Face
Below: Double-Decker

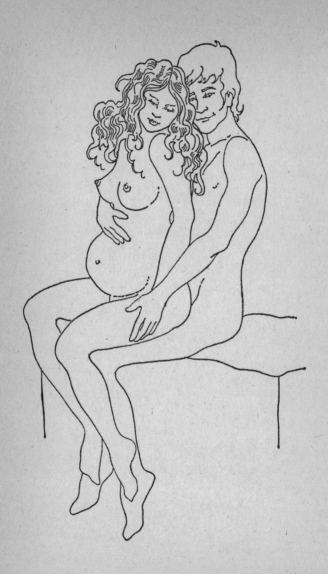

Lap Love

Ride-a-Cock-Horse

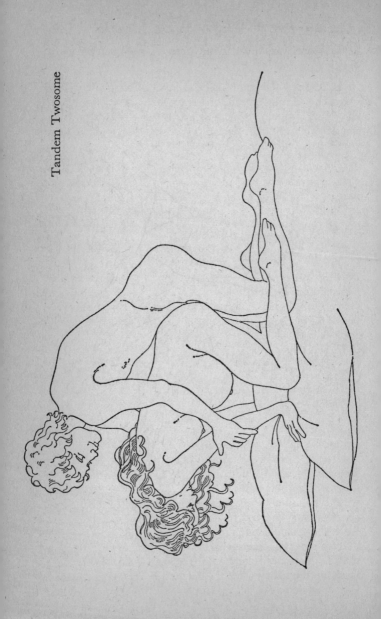

Tandem Twosome

heavy. Otherwise, the man may find it's too much like hard work!

No 4 Lap-love: The man sits on a comfortable chair, or the edge of a bed. His lady sits on his lap facing away from him. His hands are free to increase her pleasure. This position can be used right to the end of pregnancy as long as the man and the chair are both strong enough!

No 5 Ride-a-cock-horse: The man lies flat on his back. The woman sits astride him taking her weight on her knees and buttocks. The beauty of this position is that the couple face each other, and both can have their hands free. In the later stages of pregnancy when a woman feels very bulky she may be more comfortable resting more of her weight on her hands placed either side of her man's shoulders.

No 6 Tandem twosome: The woman kneels on the bed resting her weight on her hands. The man kneels upright behind her. He can use his hands to support her or to caress her. This position is fine right throughout pregnancy and is especially comfortable in the late months – in fact, it's exciting any time, pregnant or not!

Sex Problems in Pregnancy

The big worry for most couples is that intercourse may cause a miscarriage. As we've already shown in Chapter 3, a normally healthy woman doesn't have to worry about this because love-making will actually protect her pregnancy. But doctors usually advise any woman with a history of miscarriage to avoid intercourse when the second and third periods would have been due. At all other times loving can continue except, of course, if she suffers any pain or bleeding. Then she should contact her doctor immediately.

Even when miscarriage isn't a worry it's always wise for a man to avoid deep penetration, especially during the final weeks of pregnancy when the baby's head becomes engaged in the pelvic bowl.

During love-making you may occasionally feel strong contractions triggered by an orgasm. Don't worry about them. They won't harm your baby. And they won't induce labour – unless the baby is ready to be born. (So if your baby is overdue and your doctor wants to induce you, take our tip: have a lovely love-in. It's a far nicer way to persuade your baby to appear than a hospital induction.)

Tiredness is probably likely to interfere with your sex life more than anything else. And it could be aggravated by sleeplessness which affects a large number of women during pregnancy. The only way to beat it seems obvious – get more rest.

Spend a whole day or even a weekend in bed, if you can. (Get a pile of glossy magazines, borrow a portable television and you may want to spend the rest of your life pregnant.)

When tiredness, or any other problem, reduces a woman's sex drive how can she keep her loving man happy? Cuddling close may be enough for you, but you must understand that your man needs more. And loving couples can always find ways for both to reach a climax without actual intercourse.

But sometimes it's not the woman who's the reluctant lover. Many men worry about making love to a pregnant lady. First, they are afraid that by deep penetration they'll somehow damage the baby. Remember, they don't have much knowledge of a woman's pelvic anatomy! (And many don't want to know.) So they have only a hazy idea of where the baby lies and how well protected she is.

Dr. Bischoff explains: 'Worrying about hurting the baby during intercourse is very common. The man may say he's afraid of damaging the baby in some way. But what he's really afraid of, however subconsciously, is damaging his penis.'

The other great fear for men is that the baby will take all your love away from him. Too much time devoted to *your* coming baby without involving him will increase this fear. (So read our suggestions for involving him right from the start on page 25). Your man not only needs constant reassurance that he's the number one love in your life, but proof that he's passionately wanted as a lover. One of our friends who was in this spot told her man: 'I can always have another baby, but where could I find another man like you?' If this seems slushy, she argues: 'You can never tell the person you love too often how important he is to you. When you think you may be overdoing it, you're just beginning to get through!' Wiping out such jealous feelings is important because it means a man does not look on his baby as a threat to his position. And with the right attitude he'll be a more loving father right from the start.

How to Have a Sexier Pregnancy

- While you're pregnant put away any prim, high-necked nightgowns or any made of stiff fabrics. Treat yourself to nighties that are sensuous to the touch and cut low to show off your softly curving cleavage. So when your guy accidentally brushes up against you or turns over in bed he'll feel your slippery, satiny shape beside him. You may be a lot of lady but every inch will feel gorgeous!

- Surprise him – by whispering something very private in a very public place. By dropping a pile of cushions on the floor (preferably in front of a glowing fireplace) as an irresistible invitation. Or make his favourite fantasy come true by going to bed wearing just a black velvet ribbon around your throat like Goya's Maya nude – or in just a pair of silky black stockings.

- Create a sensual mood with music to make you want each other. You could try Donna Summer's classic arouser, *Love To Love You Baby*, almost any Isaac Hayes album, especially the track *Body Language*, the sexiest of oldies *Je T'Aime* by Jane Birkin and her lover Serge Gainsbourg, or any song which is specially meaningful to you both. (What you need is not singing so much as heavy breathing!)

● When you feel like spending the day in bed turn off the telephone, lock the doors and leave the world outside your bedroom door. Prepare a picnic dinner and a vacuum flask full of cold wine. Then idle away the hours in the laziest, lovingest way you know.

● Make love in the sunshine. Warm sunlight seems to pour a golden brightness over summertime lovers that makes an exciting contrast to nights in bed. Whether you try it outdoors or at home with the sun streaming through a window depends on your sense of adventure and ingenuity.

Last Minute Love-Making

Lovers will always find a way to keep on loving even when doctors ban actual intercourse. And some doctors do think that sex should stop during the last six weeks. Usually there are two reasons for this: first, they suspect that intercourse could lead to an infection. And secondly, they believe that if a woman has an orgasm it could trigger contractions which may induce an early labour.

This kind of thinking seems outdated now. If couples want to make love how can anyone stop them? And the world famous sex-doctors Masters and Johnson report that infections as a result of love-making are not more likely to occur during pregnancy. And, if you should catch an infection, which would be unusual, antibiotics could cure it quickly. So this is no longer a real problem.

As for orgasm starting labour, no one in Britain or anywhere else has proved this yet. Rosamond Bischoff says: 'After 40 years experience as a gynaecologist I believe that any labour which started after intercourse would have begun anyway.'

So healthy expectant mums can make love as much as they like, as late as they like. Medical students still smirk about the legendary couple who kept an ambulance waiting while they had a last fling before becoming parents. (We don't recommend this, incidentally.)

At this late stage many women simply don't feel sexy. And if this is your reaction, don't worry. It's not surprising when you're more sleepy, irritable and bulky. Turning over or just moving about in bed becomes difficult, so any fancy frolics are definitely out.

But with a little care and a lot of love couples can still gain plenty of satisfaction. This may range from heavy petting to what Dr. Alex Comfort calls 'Mouth Music' (oral sex).[4]

You can both gain full enjoyment with little effort in this way. Various kinds of nuzzling, nibbling, kissing and caressing intimate parts of the body come naturally to most people. And in late pregnancy the most comfortable way to enjoy them is with the woman lying on her back and her man kneeling above her. Taking turns with solo performances, the man first pleasing his lady, then she turning all her attention to him may be better now than a duet.

Sometimes a woman who has lost interest in sex may find this a wonderful way to keep her man satisfied without wanting the same in return. To a man this is 'one of the most moving gestures in the whole sexual experience'.

You may be very tired at bedtime and feel interested only in sleep. At this time, as at any other, love play is important in arousing a lady. And her man's skill in this area can make the most tired expectant mother suddenly feel wide-awake. Often, a woman may start by just enjoying the closeness of intercourse without wanting a climax. But the warmth of his gentle loving may set her alight.

The way to keep your relationship satisfying right to the end is to let your man do most of the work, especially in actual intercourse. But a tender, experimental shot-in-the-dark may prove surprisingly delicious. Together you can work out some lovely new melodies to add to your repertoire of loving.

CHAPTER SEVEN

If You've Got It, Flaunt It

Here they come . . . the marvellous middle months of pregnancy. This is the stage when your body begins to reward you for staggering through those nauseous first months. It's almost like getting an enormous transfusion of vitality. You feel you've never looked or felt better. Your love life zings – and it shows.

Most women find that they feel sexier now than at any time in their lives. That's the finding of sex therapists Masters and Johnson. They discovered that most of the women they studied not only had stronger sex drives – but also had more love-making fantasies, more erotic dreams and wanted wilder performances in bed. This applied to women whether pregnant for the first time or the ninth![1]

Your fella will also have a wonderful time now getting to know his new luscious lady. Suddenly he has his hands full with a super-feminine woman. Around the sixteenth week he'll notice that your bosom is firmer and fuller. Girls who've always longed for a curvy cleavage find they have one at last. And even big bosomed ladies love their taut new shape.

This is all part of the celebrated bloom of pregnancy. The lovely difference in your outline is the result of the wonderful changes inside your body. Your heart is pumping out 40 per cent more blood and this is richer now, carrying more nourishment for you and your baby. So your eyes shine, your hair gets glossier, your nails lengthen and strengthen. Your complexion is clearer, smoother. And all over your body the skin has a creamy softness just like a ripe peach. You look and feel delicious!

Why not exploit your glowing good looks? If you've never done it before buy a dress with a softly revealing neckline. When you've an over-flowing cleavage we guarantee no one will notice a thickening waistline. Your motto should be: if you've got it, flaunt it – and that includes a 40-inch bustline!

And if you want to heighten the sweet appeal of bare skin take a tip from top photographic models. Before stepping in front of the cameras they always smooth a dab of baby oil on to their breasts. This adds a satiny polish to the skin which has an enticing look, especially in soft evening light. Less messy but equally effective is transparent face gloss.

You'll also begin to notice now that the early tenderness and tingling discomfort in your breasts has disappeared. But they are still quite sensitive. So although they need gentle handling in love-play the sensations you get from them should be doubly erotic now. This is also the time when one part of your beauty care – massaging cream into your breasts and body – can be a sensuous experience for both you and your man. If he lends a hand it could lead to more than a beauty treatment.

Every woman should take advantage of the special charm of firm curves and blooming skin. They bring a soft allure even to the plainest face and figure.

You may find it hard to believe that a girl whose vital statistics are 40–40–40 can turn on the opposite sex. Well, you're in for a beautiful surprise! A lot of men find pregnant women very attractive. That's the verdict of psychologist Jane Firbank who explains: 'The reason is the sexual tension that usually exists between men and women disappears. The pregnant woman doesn't have to prove herself to every man she meets. After all, she's conceived already. So it's obvious she has a mate and isn't looking for one. You notice the same behaviour in a girl who's just engaged. She relaxes around other men because she has the proof that she belongs to just one man. Well, pregnancy is the ultimate proof that you are one man's woman.'

Dr. Alex Comfort suspects that there's a more subtle

secret of a pregnant woman's appeal to men. He believes that her body may give off a special subliminal scent called a pheromone.

The body does give off these scents at various times. Consciously we can't detect them but we react to them nevertheless. Research with animals shows that pheromones play a powerful role in attracting male animals to the female of the species, especially at mating times. Maybe this sub-conscious attraction works for the human female, too, while she is pregnant.

Pheromones may be the secret of surprises like this one: a girl who was six months pregnant went to meet her husband for a drink in a television company's club. A gorgeous cameraman who knew her slightly, saw her, stopped and said: 'You look fantastic!' He insisted on buying her a bottle of champagne and kept the compliments flowing until her husband arrived to take her home. This lady says she norm-ally never gets a second glance from other men. Needless to say, she is now thinking of becoming pregnant again.

In the company of a pregnant woman nearly all men become much more attentive and courteous. (It's practically the only time you'll be offered a seat in a crowded bus or train – so enjoy it!) It's a beautiful experience for both you and the man. He'll love spoiling you every bit as much as you do.

Many husbands are surprised by the extra warmth between their pregnant wives and their men friends. But these friendships rarely threaten a happy marriage and a clever girl treats each man she meets like her very own Sir Galahad. We found that even hard-bitten newspapermen who can usually never bother to lift their eyes from their headlines made us feel special when we were pregnant. They actually looked up from their pints in the pub, grinned and said: 'Hello, Fatso!'

But not only men are attracted to pregnant ladies. Women and children become much friendlier, too. Even people who aren't close pals seems to have no hesitation about patting, stroking or hugging an expectant mum. And sometimes only slight acquaintances will give your stomach a friendly pat or ask to feel the baby moving.

Have you ever watched people in the sculpture gallery of a museum examining a beautiful work of art? And seen the look on their faces as their hands flow over its rhythmic curves? The same wonder and admiration is on your friend's faces when they stroke your bulging tummy. It's almost as if your body was a beautiful, curving sculpture, too. You're irresistible!

And the reason people take such liberties? It's body language. We all give off subconscious signals to other people with every glance, every movement, every word. A woman who slips easily into the physical changes of pregnancy may have a relaxed open appeal to others. Her voice is softer, calmer. She smiles often and the lines of her figure are more relaxed. Her body language says: 'Look at my figure! Isn't it wonderful!' And anyone who comes within range of this happy message can't fail to agree.

When her figure returns to normal a woman finds that these caresses and little courtesies suddenly stop. So make the most of them while they last.

The First High

The moment you first feel your baby moving inside you is one of every expectant mother's biggest thrills. This usually happens on average between the 16th and 20th weeks. (In a first pregnancy you can expect these soft flutterings between 18 and 24 weeks; in a second or subsequent pregnancy the gentle movements arrive sooner, around 16 weeks or more rarely about the 14th week.

The sensation is rather like being tickled on the inside with the fronds of a feather. Or just like your stomach turning over with excitement. Some women mistake the feeling for an unromantic attack of wind! And it may be a month or so at least before these faint flutterings are strong enough to be noticed by anyone else. But most first time fathers will be keen to feel them. For many men this is the big occasion when their baby begins to be real. Suddenly it is a little independent being, stretching, tossing, and turning somersaults.

Sharing the excitement of feeling the stirrings of their unborn child is one more way in which pregnancy can bind lovers even closer together. But don't be too upset if your man is one of those who does not want to be so closely involved. Many fathers are freaked by the knowledge that they will soon be responsible for a new person. And they also may subconsciously feel resentful when their wives are obviously thinking of little else but the new arrival. So they feel left out. And at this stage, remember that fathers are not really concerned with the progress of your pregnancy. So this is where a perceptive wife will give her man a lot more attention, realising that this is only a phase that soon passes.

Inflation Fashion

Fashion today is free and fun, sexy and sporty – in fact, anything you want it to be. And whatever your style of dressing there's no need to change it just because you're pregnant.

But before you splurge on maternity fashions for inflated figures, think about the following points:

1 *Don't wear maternity clothes too soon.* You're probably longing to tell the world your good news by showing off your changed outline. But if you start wearing loose, smocky dresses before you *really* need them you'll be bored with them all long before your nine months ends. So wear your normal clothes as long as you possibly can.

2 *Don't buy too many maternity clothes.* If a special occasion comes up you don't have to splurge on a roomy party dress. You can always hire one for a nominal cost. Your local branch of the National Childbirth Trust may help

here. Also watch for Rent-A-Tent advertisements in the local press.

3 *You don't have to buy clothes in maternity boutiques.* Many loose-fitting styles for ordinary girls can be comfortably worn by an expectant mum. But for comfort remember you'll need one size larger around the bustline.

4 *Avoid dresses and tops in stiff fabrics.* Soft materials which flow gently around your figure look less bulky and more appealing.

5 *Why look frumpy in drab colours and high-necked styles?* Dark colours may be hard-wearing and practical but spicier shades will do more for your looks. Dare to be a little revealing. A lower neckline will draw attention away from your mountainous waistline. Pay lots of attention to your grooming with well-shaped nails, clean, shiny hair and soft, pretty make-up.

In summer ordinary tee-shirts can be worn under loose-fitting pinafore dresses. But if you want one dress which will take you through a change of seasons choose one in denim. This will wash and wear well, is cool enough for warm days and can be worn over a roll-necked sweater in cold weather. For a winter pregnancy a new overcoat seems an extravagance. (Most pregnant women don't feel the cold as much as other people – a baby provides portable central heating!) So a shawl or poncho may be sufficient for cooler days and is still useful after the birth.

Avoid dresses with an empire line, tightly fitted under the bosom. By the end of nine months any tightness around the bust becomes uncomfortable. And as the baby grows your ribcage expands to allow room for the top of the enlarging womb. So dresses which fall straight from the shoulder are more comfortable. Ethnic clothing stores have many styles which are particularly attractive on expectant ladies. A simple caftan is ideal, and makes a wonderful evening gown.

Jeans with expanding waistlines can be found in some big city stores and boutiques. But we think the few months they're useful doesn't justify their high price. If you must live in trousers unzip the flies and sew tapes on the front waist fastening of ordinary trousers. Or buy Indian men's drawstring pants (on which the western pyjamas is based). Then you can gradually loosen the waist as you grow, and hide the waistline with a smocky top.

By studying your new shape in a full length mirror you'll realise that your enlarging tummy has changed your proportions. Very short skirts look ridiculous and rather vulgar now. Only very young, slim girls can wear them successfully. The most flattering hemline is slightly below the knee for most girls or mid-calf for really tall girls. The extra length seems to balance your extra width.

If you are tempted to spend lots of money on clothes buy cologne instead. Few things say more about you than your scent. If it's sweet, clean-smelling and clingy you'll leave a lovely impression everywhere you go. So choose your favourite fragrance in oils, gels, bubble baths, perfume or toilet water and splash it on all day long.

During pregnancy extra care is necessary to stay fresh. A woman's natural vaginal secretions increase, especially in the early months and may become a problem. Dr. Eugene Schoenfeld, better known in the United States as Dr. Hip for his frank advice on sex and health, says: 'I think there is no finer odour than a healthy woman's smell. It's sexually attractive. There was a time in history when women applied a handkerchief to the vagina then wore it on the shoulder as a sexual lure.'

But he warns this fresh tantalising smell may soon become offensive. 'It's especially important for women not to wear synthetic underwear or any impermeable fabric. Any fabric that doesn't allow air circulation changes the ecology of the vagina, keeps it hot and moist, and encourages the growth of bacteria.' Cool, porous cotton, he feels, is therefore better to wear than non-porous nylon or other synthetic materials. So during pregnancy stick to cotton underwear. Avoid sealing off your body from waist to feet in nylon tights, knickers and slips. You'll not only feel more comfortable in cotton (or silk if your bank account runs to such treats!) but you'll keep your after-bath freshness longer. And when you wear tights buy the crotch-less kind in a very large size.

The Rhythm of Life

Never do you feel the rhythm of life more powerfully than when you give birth. It's a rare and thrilling event in any woman's life. So it seems a pity that many people link child-birth with fear and pain. They don't realise that only 30 per cent of labour is the sheer physical hard work of pushing a baby out into the world. The remaining 70 per cent is the emotional experience that you undergo.

This is a clear example of mind over matter. What you *believe* is more significant than what you *feel*. And it's the reason relaxation classes are essential for every mother-to-be. We know from our own experiences that preparing your mind fully for delivery day makes it easier on your body.

The most popular method today is a technique called 'psychoprophylaxis', an invented word which, according to its first British promoter, Erna Wright, means 'prevention through the mind'. The whole idea is to stop pain before it starts by using your mind to control your muscles.

All this sounds far more complicated than it actually is. Women who go to psychoprophylaxis classes learn to do a series of breathing exercises which help their muscles to relax. As the womb is one of the few muscles we cannot control, these exercises, done during labour, allow the womb to do its work without other muscles in the body tensing up and using energy the womb needs to deliver the baby. By preventing these other muscles from slowing up the whole birth process these exercises help you to have a shorter, easier labour. And surely that's what every woman wants? What's more, because they enable you to stay in control you can be alert and aware of every exciting minute. In fact, you're likely to enjoy the experience of birth, rather than getting lost in waves of continuous pain.

The first mother trained to use these relaxation methods gave birth to a baby in Russia in 1949. Today, there are many thousands of classes to teach this method around the world. In Britain they are usually run by local authorities, through maternity hospitals or groups backed by the National Childbirth Trust.

But are these relaxation classes really effective in reducing pain? From many thousands of labour reports sent to the National Childbirth Trust from ex-pupils, they reckon that 30 per cent of all pregnant women who are trained in the relaxation method have a much easier labour because mothers have been taught exactly how to cope with contractions. And gynaecologist Derek Llewellyn-Jones says that 45 per cent of all women who use this method need no other pain reliever. Only one in 100 finds it doesn't work at all. Says a Trust teacher: 'Even if it helps only psychologically, that's better than nothing.'

When you do these special breathing exercises you learn to distract your mind from the pain of a contraction. Instead of tensing up when it happens you allow the natural rhythms of your body to take over. So each contraction flows over your belly like a wave, always helping labour, never hindering it. At the classes you also learn exercises like the pelvic rock which help with backache in the later stages of pregnancy and during labour. They teach you the right way to push out the baby, and just as important, the right moment to start pushing.

To make childbirth less of an ordeal you need to know what's happening to your body and be prepared for it. Relaxation classes do all this. Which is the reason we think they're essential. An extra advantage of learning to breathe correctly is that these exercises, like yoga, help you through *any* stressful situation in life. They calm the mind, banish tension and so you are better able to cope.

When you go to your first ante-natal clinic, ask for the address of the nearest relaxation classes. If none is available in your area, contact the National Childbirth Trust (*see* Useful Addresses, page 263).

Don't worry that if you start your labour with relaxation techniques, you can't combine them with other pain-relieving methods offered by the hospital. As keen as we both are on relaxation classes, we feel you should take advantage of any painkiller you find necessary, without worrying that you have 'failed'. Everyone can tolerate different amounts of pain because we are all sensitive to different degrees. So don't blame yourself if you want something extra to help you have a better labour. (We discuss all available pain relievers on page 123 so you can make a fully informed choice.)

We don't want to gloss over the fact that labour is damned hard work and often very painful. Even when it's relatively easy it's no picnic and we can think of a dozen different ways to spend a day that are better than being in labour – such as having all your teeth extracted without anaesthetic!

CHAPTER EIGHT

Kitting Out The Kid

One of the earliest symptoms of pregnancy is a mad urge to spend money. We know of girls, little more than seconds pregnant, who bought complete layettes on the way home from their first visit to the doctor!

Babies are big business these days because shops make money out of those motherly urges. It's no accident that since the Seventies began almost every high street seems to have a chain store devoted to the needs of babies. But every time you go shopping for your expected baby remember that newborns don't care what they wear, feel just as warm in hand-me-downs as new clothes, and can't tell the difference between genuine antiques and junk store bargains.

All this doesn't mean we think your kid should be kitted out cheapo-cheapo style. But if your budget can't stretch as far as you'd like it to, remember this: babies shoot up faster than Jack's beanstalk. A ton of barely-worn baby wear is great only for baby firms' profits but rotten for your bank balance.

Okay, you want your child to look gorgeous and dazzle every visitor. But so much second-hand, only slightly used equipment such as cots and prams is available that no one would guess you didn't buy all new stuff. Just look at your local newspaper's small ads section and you'll see endless bargains, from high chairs to low chairs, from bouncers to strollers. All cut price and mostly in beautiful condition. Other places to watch for bargains are notice boards at your local baby clinic, 'For Sale' cards in your nearest newsagent's window, and at relaxation classes.

Apart from gifts from doting grannies none of the equipment we had for our babies was brand new – proving that we practise what we preach! So here are two lists of the articles you really need and the spend-traps to avoid.

Basic Equipment for Newborns

What to buy   *And why*

Two buckets with lids: For soaking damp and dirty nappies. Save money by avoiding the fancy, flowered pails in pretty colours. Buy plain ones and add transfers if you must.

Long-handled white plastic brewing spoon: You can find this in the home brew section of your chemist or hardware store. Use it for stirring nappies in sterilising solution (*see* Chapter 17).

Washing machine (preferably automatic):   Some people don't think this is essential. But we would have slit our throats, ankles and wrists without one. Unless you live on top of a launderette, your own machine is a fantastic time and energy saver.

Nursing chair: For comfort at feeding times. Any low, armless chair with a firm back will do. You don't want to add backache to the tiredness you'll feel as a new mum. Comb junk shops, jumble sales for a good buy. Add a

	stretch cover or coat of paint if necessary.
Baby mobile:	Bored babies cry. But a mobile will keep her happy for hours. (*See* Chapter 18.)
Cat net:	Never leave a baby alone outdoors without a fine net covering the pram. Apart from birds and animals it also protects your baby from insects and falling leaves.
Chest of drawers:	Don't buy dinky, teeny-sized drawers. The number of clothes a baby owns grows as fast as she does. And you'll always need extra storage space. So buy the largest chest you can comfortably fit into the baby's room. Become a jumble sale or junk shop scavenger. Be prepared to strip or paint your bargain.
Something to sleep in, like a carry-cot:	This can double as a pram. It is compact, may be left on table tops. Doesn't take up much room even in a bedsitter. A model is now available which converts from carry-cot to pram to stroller. This saves both money and space.
Cot-sized cellular blanket:	Bedclothes for newborns must be lightweight yet warm. A cot-sized blanket can be folded in four to fit a crib or carry-cot.

	Later, it's one less blanket to buy for the cot.
3 or 4 cot-sized sheets:	Again, fold them in half to fit the carry-cot. Later, you'll need all these sheets when the baby moves into a cot. An old single-bed sheet divided makes two generous-sized cot sheets.
Changing table (approx. 2 ft. 6 ins. × 4 ft.):	A sturdy, waist-high table is essential for dressing, changing and bathing a baby if you want to avoid backache. Don't worry if you have a weather-beaten one. Just cover the top with stick-on vinyl. This table will be ideal later for young artists and homework.
Changing mat:	A padded, plastic-covered mat. This cushions the baby against lying on a hard surface during nappy changes. Cover it with a nappy to prevent the baby's skin touching cold plastic. The mat wipes clean, costs only a few pounds new and much less second-hand. (Using your lap to change new-borns is fine, but this gets dodgy later with larger, more active babies.)
2 medium-sized soft pile towels:	Buy them in bright colours, not insipid pastels.

Equipment for Older Babies

Stroller: collapsible fold-away pushchair with plastic rain-cover:

For use when the baby is six months old or can sit unsupported. Don't, repeat *do not* put a younger baby into a push-chair. The soft back cannot support a very young spine and may actually harm your baby. Best of all is a firm-backed stroller, unfortunately these are not completely foldaway. But which is better – a healthy spine or a convenient baby carriage?

A drop-side cot:

You won't need a cot until the baby is around 4 months old, so you have plenty of time to look for a good, second-hand one.

High-chair with safety harness:

For use when the baby can sit up. Once again look for a second-hand money-saver. The simpler the design the easier it is to clean. Nooks and fancy crannies collect grime and food. Most high-chairs convert into a low chair and table. The safety harness will prevent accidents.

Safety bath mat:

This lines the bottom of the bath and prevents the baby slipping over. For use when the baby switches to bathing in the family tub at around 5 months.

Baby clothes to buy	*And why*
Two dozen best quality towelling nappies:	Top quality nappies are essential because they must withstand two years of soaking, washing and drying.
6 safety nappy pins:	Buy famous brands' seconds which have reduced prices only because of slight flaws. (*See* Chapter 17.)
Three pairs elastic-waisted plastic pants (newborn size): 1 packet tie-on plastic pants:	To make baby's bottom waterproof. Plastic pants save a lot of work for mum but have one drawback. They can prevent air circulating around the nappy, thus keeping it moist. Tie-on pants are more airy though not leakproof overnight. (*See* Chapter 17.)
6 vests:	For a winter baby, four should be of fine wool and two in cotton. A summer baby needs the reverse, two wool, four cotton. The vests should have envelope-style necks which open to slide over a baby's head then close up again snugly.
4 stretch sleepsuits (0–3 months size, or nightgowns for summer babies):	One to wear, one in the wash and two at the ready.
2 jackets or cardigans:	To wear inside the house in cold weather. Or for trips outside under a shawl or blanket.

2 bonnets:	Bonnets and mittens are essential in cool weather as a newborn baby loses body heat rapidly, especially from its disproportionately large head. Buy one bonnet larger than the other.
2 pairs mittens:	

Shawl or blanket:　　　　　To keep the baby warm on outings or in draughty rooms.

Baby Beauty Aids to buy　　*And why*

(for bottoms)

Cotton wool on a roll:	For wiping bottoms clean. Also for use cleaning faces, ears and nose. Don't waste money on more expensive cotton wool balls. You can tear off little lumps from a roll.
Baby lotion or oil: (largest size)	Kinder for nappy rash than soap and water.
1 giant-size jar zinc and castor oil cream:	Softens, protects and waterproofs the baby's skin against damp nappies.
Disposable nappy liners:	How did mums ever live without them? Make soiled nappies easier to handle. Just drop the dirty liner down the lavatory and it flushes away. The nappy will be left relatively clean. (*See* Chapter 17.)
Nappy steriliser:	No need to buy expensive famous brands when you can

easily make your own with ordinary household bleach. (*See* Chapter 17.)

(for tops)

Baby soap:

Any pure, super-fatted soap sold by chemists is fine. We do NOT recommend detergent-style soap for babies. The fewer chemicals which come into contact with baby skin the better.

Talcum powder:

Not essential but makes sweet-smelling babies. Make sure the skin is absolutely dry before applying. Don't sprinkle it on nappy area because it clogs up in creases and irritates the skin between the legs. Don't sprinkle near a baby's face as it shouldn't be inhaled.

Hairbrush:

A musical brush makes a baby enjoy haircare, and can also be used as a rattle.

Feeding Equipment

Even if you breast feed you need at least two feeding bottles for your baby's drinks of water and orange juice.

What to buy	*And why*
8 wide-necked feeding bottles, plastic not glass:	The wide-necked ones are much easier to clean.

8 matching teats: (small-hole size)	For newborns. (Bottles are usually sold complete with teats, caps, etc.)
Sterilising box large enough to hold 8 bottles immersed in water:	Any large plastic box approx. 2 feet by $1\frac{1}{2}$ feet and about 8–10 inches deep, such as a plastic breadbin, will do the job. Make sure the box has a lid. Metal won't do because it corrodes. China or glass is fine if not chipped. The box will be useful later for storage when the baby no longer has bottles.
Sterilising liquid or tablets:	For hygienically soaking bottles, teats, caps and other feeding equipment.
Bottle brush:	For cleaning bottles before sterilising.
Plastic knife:	For levelling off scoops of baby milk powder before mixing bottle feeds. Must be plastic as metal corrodes in steriliser.
Plastic strainer:	For straining orange juice so that it flows freely through a teat. An ordinary coffee strainer will do.
Small washing-up brush:	For scrubbing teats, bottle caps and other feeding equipment. Must be used only for this purpose.

Optional Extras

Disposable nappies:
For use when you're too tired to wash and dry a load of towelling nappies, or on day trips when you don't want to carry soiled nappies about. Buy in bulk if possible. Also handy used with a towelling nappy to make it more absorbent overnight.

Moist medicated baby wipes:
Ideal for cleaning bottoms, hands and face when travelling. Or in an emergency at home. Not recommended for use at every nappy change. Constant use may cause a rash. Damp cotton wool is cheaper and kinder to sensitive baby skin.

Rigid-backed baby chair:
As soon as your baby begins to notice the world around her she will enjoy sitting propped up in one of these chairs which give good support and have safety straps to stop her falling out. Most are available with extra attachments for converting into a high chair or swing. We think you need only the basic chair. Watch for a good, second-hand buy.

Disposable pre-sterilised feeding bootles:
If you're worried about sterilising and cleaning bottles properly these are the solution. They cost more than ordinary bottles but are easy and safe to use.

Ideal for travelling when sterilising isn't easy.

Sleeping bag: This fits inside a carry-cot and makes transporting the baby easy and snug. It's lightweight and washable.

Baby Goods You Don't Need

Don't buy   *And why*

Bottle warmers: If you can get your baby accustomed to bottles almost straight from the fridge it's far more hygienic. Heating bottles makes germs multiply.

Shaped nappies: An unnecessary extravagance. They are pricey and do the same job as ordinary towelling squares.

Fancy frilled crib: If you can borrow one or get one as a gift, fine. Otherwise a new crib is a waste of money. The baby will grow out of it in three or four months.

Changing unit: Unsuitable for any other purpose, takes up space. Does not hold as many clothes as a chest of drawers.

Bath stands or canvas baths: You don't need a bath stand or other equipment because you can easily bath the baby in a hand basin or kitchen sink. If you are given a baby bath you can stand it on a table.

Wardrobe: Not necessary until your child is over a year old.

Baby weighing scales: You can weigh your baby as often as you like at the baby health clinic. Some clinics will lend you scales for a 24 hour test of weight.

Pram canopies, parasols: On many prams you can tilt the hood to keep off the sun. When the baby is old enough to sit in a stroller use a sunhat.

On every item of baby equipment you buy look for the British Standards number which is your guarantee of safety. Here are the numbers for each article.

Dummies	BS 5239	Car seats	BS 3254
Wooden cots	BS 1753	or	BS AU 157A
Cot mattresses	BS 1877	Toys	BS 3443
Fireguards	BS 3140	Harnesses	BS 3785
Carry-cots	BS 3881	Medicine chests	BS 3922
Pushchairs	BS 4792	Safety barriers	BS 4125

Super Sanity-Savers

Baby sling: A crying baby will soon be soothed when held close to a mother's heart in a sling. Useful in those desperate hours when the baby is shrieking, you have to cook supper and there's someone knocking at the front door. Of course, it's also an ideal way to carry a baby too young for a stroller.

Judy: 'I used to go shopping looking like a pregnant womble two months after my daughter was born. Wrapped inside my coat my baby rode snugly close to my chest. On a bitter winter day she was far warmer than if she had been wheeled around in a pram. And she was happier being right up close to me. (*See* Chapter 19.)

Bulk buying: Buy as many items as you can from baby lotion to bottom wipes in the largest economy sizes you can find in shops or discount stores. The main advantage of this is not the small saving in money, it's the time-saving convenience. Discovering you are about to run out of nappy liners on a snowy day in those first tiring weeks is enough to make you take an overdose of gripewater.

Antiseptic talc: At the hospital you'll usually be given a small tin of this talcum to help in drying up the stub of the baby's umbilical cord. Take the tin home with you because it's also useful for healing little spots on baby skin.

Sedatives: Don't be shy about asking your health visitor or doctor about a sedative for the baby if she is driving you crazy at night for no apparent reason. (*See* Chapter 18.) The doctor may prescribe a mild sedative which will get your baby into the habit of sleeping longer at night. Nothing wrecks the joys of motherhood more than lack of sleep.

Teething powders and gels: Sometimes these are effective, sometimes they're not. If they work, fine. If not, keep singing those lullabies.

Label your pram: In these mass-production days when identical prams and strollers are left outside super-markets or clinics how can you tell which one is yours?

Judy: 'My two-day-old pushchair left in a bus baggage section was swiped by an unscrupulous mum who left behind her old, tatty version of the same model. What this nasty thief didn't know when she took my sparkling new baby carriage was the previous day 1 had buckled one of the wheels on an escalator. You may spot her when she wheels a wobbling buggy down your street.'

Sure cure for sick smells: Dilute bicarbonate of soda with water and use this solution to clean anything a baby has sicked up on. The nasty smell of vomit will vanish instantly. And this is safe to use on any surface, even hair and skin. Wonderful for car sickness on long journeys. And add some to the washing machine when laundering clothes covered in sick.

Val: 'I was giving Judy and her baby Jordan a lift in my Mini when, for no reason, Jordan suddenly threw up. Both the child and the back of the car were covered. When we got home, I attended to the baby while Judy tackled the car. She sprinkled liberal quantities of bicarb into a bucket of hot water and washed the car thoroughly while I changed Jordan and washed her hair and hands with a solution of water and bicarb. Her clothes went into the washing machine, again sprinkled with more bicarb. After this furious activity, there was not even a trace of the smell. Not in the car and not on the small body and neither seem the worse for the adventure.'

Present Time

Most new mums are showered with gifts. But a great many of these presents will never be used, simply because they're either impractical or disliked. Some of the goodies we received from well-meaning relatives and friends never came out of their wrappings. These included a pink plastic fish with a thermometer for a spine (intended for gauging the right heat for baby's bathwater, but your elbow can do the same job), a plastic bottle with a spoon attachment for splurging baby's first mixed feeds on to the spoon by squeezing the bottle; Swansdown booties that looked bedraggled after the first wash; 2 million matinee jackets with frilly bows all of which wouldn't survive one trip through the washing machine, (and who has time for hand washing?); deliciously pretty sets of embroidered baby pillowcases which remained unused because babies should not sleep with pillows until around the age of two, if then.

As there are countless gadgets mums crave but can't afford it seems a pity friends don't give you exactly what you need. The most tactful way to get them to do this may be to steal an idea from brides, and produce a list of the gifts you really would use, then leave it discreetly with a sympathetic close friend who can circulate it for you. Here are our suggestions to add to your list.

A month's supply of disposable nappies

A baby bath (if you have enough space for one)

A polo-necked baby poncho, prettier and warmer than a cardigan or jacket in winter, fits all size babies and is not so quickly outgrown as a coat

Any clothes for an older baby because newborn sizes last only a few weeks

A rose or fruit tree to plant in the garden and compare its growth with your child

A baby sling

Fun pyjamas or nightgowns in sizes up to 18 months

A laundry basket to keep soiled baby clothes separate from the family wash

Baby china such as a cereal bowl, plate or cup

Sunbonnet or sun hat

A patchwork or crocheted quilt for pram or cot

Rag dolls, bath toys, brightly coloured, tinkling mobiles

A smart mother's hold-all for carrying nappies, etc. on visits

Any educational toy

A mirror decorated with children's transfers

A set of baby's first books to encourage an early appreciation of reading

A photographic album to record the baby's progress

A music box or jack-in-the-box

A Baby Bouncer – bouncing seat for smaller babies, or a harness on a spring which fastens to a door frame, for 8-month-olds

CHAPTER NINE

Big Can Be Beautiful

When a tape measure goes 40 inches around your waist and you smile, you're in the last stage of pregnancy. This is the time to prove that big really can be beautiful.

A lot of women feel like bloated balloons convinced they will never see their toes again. That sort of thinking is a bring-down. You have to change your attitude to make the most of these last, loaded months. So don't think of your waist as being more than twice its normal size. Instead say to yourself: 'I'm in the Top 40 now'. Throw your weight around. Act like a pregnant superstar.

Val: 'When I was nearing the end of my pregnancy and still working, I used to run around town in my Mini and park it outside the entrance of any place I had to visit – whether parking was permissible or not. But I always took the precaution of sticking a little notice under the windscreen wiper saying: "Highly pregnant driver. Baby imminent. *Please* do not tow away". In all the time I did this I never got a ticket. But one day after I returned to my car, parked on a taxi rank, I found someone had added to my note: "We are a taxi service and also do deliveries".'

To look as proud of your curving belly as you feel, always stand and sit up straight. Never ever slouch. To see a very pregnant lady holding herself beautifully is a lovely sight. But it not only looks great, it relieves much of the extra strain on your spine. This prevents backache, one of the common hazards of pregnancy. Slumping in a chair or lounging about only increases that tired feeling. When you do have a chance to relax remember to put your feet up higher than your waist. This helps the leg veins to cope more easily with the increased demands of pregnancy.

Living with a Mountain Round your Middle

Towards the end of your 40 weeks simple things like getting out of bed can become tricky. 20 pounds of baby bump around your middle tends to throw you off balance. No longer can you spring out of bed so lightly in the mornings. Our favourite gynaecologist gave us a terrific tip for lifting your extra weight easily from a prone position to an upright one.

First, loosen the blankets. Have a really good kick, wriggle and stretch. All your muscles are warming up. Your circulation gets into gear. Take a few deep breaths. Then while still lying down turn your hips slightly in a swivelling movement towards the direction you are going to get out of bed. Swing both legs over the side of the bed. Then roll over on your side on the edge of the bed until your feet can touch the floor. Now, use your arms to level yourself into a standing position. This will prevent pins and needles, one of the commonest complaints of pregnancy. We know one sufferer who sprained her ankle when she tried to get out of bed and put all her weight on her legs too quickly.

A lot of pregnant women avoid stairs and take lifts or escalators whenever possible. Don't! Climbing stairs is great exercise. It stretches the hip joints – especially if you go up them two at a time holding on to the bannister. To get any benefit out of this exercise you must go slowly and steadily. It's even better if you climb the stairs on all fours like a monkey. Sounds ridiculous but it really helps to give you loose muscles, and so an easier labour.

Coming down stairs is different. Never, never walk downstairs carrying a heavy weight like a basket of shopping or a toddler. If no one else is around to help you here's the routine: leave the bundle at the top of the stairs. Walk down three steps, then sit down. Reach back for the bundle and bring it down to your level. Keep repeating this until you reach ground level.

Shopping is something else that needs planning. Usually though, friends or relatives may do some for you, but there's always a certain amount you have to do yourself. Before you set out sit down and make a list. Work out the easiest route through your shopping centre to avoid back-tracking and unnecessary walking. The earlier in the morning you go shopping the better. Your body collects fluid throughout the day. So you will feel at your heaviest and least active in the late afternoon.

If you have to shop with a toddler you probably need twice as much planning before and rest afterwards. It's not impossible to rest with a small, active child. around, just *nearly* impossible. So you must be cunning. We believe that parents have rights too. But only sneaky parents ever get to exercise those rights. So if you need a rest and there's an energetic 2-year-old bopping around your ankles, the superior cunning you're supposed to have should out-manoeuvre the smartest toddler.

If your kid is whining she's probably bored. So let her feel helpful by doing little jobs for you. One mum we know used to do embroidery while resting. She wore out her pestering 3-year-old son by sending him upstairs first to get the red wool, then the blue, then the green and so on, until he was tired enough for an early nap. Other ideas to keep a small person entertained include a treasure hunt around the house searching for unshelled peanuts, building blocks or spare, shiny buttons from your sewing basket.

Rearranging your pots and pans is noisy. It's always worth a try though and so is playing statues: make her sit or lie very still and watch to see if she moves as much as an eyelash. We've known this keep a small child quiet for the lengthy period of about 35 seconds. Stretch this to maybe 5 minutes by offering a small prize. When absolutely desperate try to resist the impulse to lose her while out shopping. Even if you think you'd both have a much nicer afternoon – she at the police station being gorged with ice-cream and you at home in bed!

Ten Essentials that Aren't on any Hospital's List

Many mums have been surprised by babies who decided to arrive early. So it makes sense to get all essentials for both of you well before the last few weeks of your pregnancy. Shopping for a mum who's in hospital causes a big flap among your friends and relatives – and remember, their taste may not be yours. It's better, therefore, to choose everything yourself.

Pack your suitcase for the hospital at least a month before the delivery date. You may be able to borrow a few goodies from friends, like special nightgowns, but it's nice to have at least one new, super nightie to dazzle the doctors. (If you plan to breast feed make sure all your nightgowns have front openings down to the waist.) For a 10-day hospital stay you you will need at least 3 – 1 to wear, 1 in your locker for emergencies, and 1 in the wash.

Apart from basic toilet articles like toothpaste and deodorant that you take on any trip, plus the extra items the hopsital asks you to bring, we suggest you pack the following:

1   3 boxes of paper knickers. This saves sending home soiled ones to be laundered. Having a ready, clean supply means you can change your underwear as often as you wish during the day. And those you take off go straight into the hospital's incinerator.

2   A vacuum flask for cold soft drinks or extra pintas. In the necessary heat of a maternity ward you'll build up a big thirst. And iced drinks are difficult to get in busy hospitals. The more fluids you drink the better if you plan to breast feed.

3   Writing paper, a pen, address book, and *stamps* for thank-you notes.

4   A large container of ordinary cooking salt. Liberally sprinkled in your bath water this helps to soothe and heal episiotomy stitches. 2 or 3 baths each day make you feel far more comfortable. Some hospitals do supply salt but you'd be surprised how fast it disappears.

5   2 bras with strong supporting cups (front-opening style if you plan to breast-feed. And a large box of breast pads to line the bra cups and absorb leakages of milk. (You need these even if you're bottle feeding because you'll still drip a little until your supply dries up.)

6   A large bottle of your favourite cologne to splash on and make you feel fragrant and banish the milky odour that clings to new mums. And an aerosol can of Evian water for a fresh feeling in hospital as well as during labour. The cooling spray will really help when you feel you're wilting with tiredness.

7   A box of moisturised, scented paper towels in sachets for cleaning hands and face without getting out of bed.

8   1 box of man-sized paper tissues, uses too numerous to list.

9   An extra pillow to give you back support is a boon in labour, and also useful when you sit up to see visitors. Many NHS hospitals don't have enough to go round.

10   Ear plugs to give you peace and quiet at night or during daytime naps, and block out noises and heavy breathing made by your wardmates. Buy them in a box at your chemist.

Jazzing up the Last Dreary Weeks

Too many women miss the real significance of the last weeks of pregnancy. Feeling they've been pregnant for centuries they're anxious to get the birth safely over. But by trying to speed up these last dreary, dragging weeks they forfeit a very special time, especially when expecting a first child. These are the last lovely lazy days you and your man share. Sunday morning lie-ins will soon be just a memory. So will all-night parties, taking off on trips when you feel like it, and making love exactly when you want to, not just when the baby is sleeping.

Even if you already have a toddler, after the new baby arrives you and your man will have even less time together. So exploit these last special weeks. Here are 6 super ways to brighten up the final chapter of your pregnancy.

1   Organise a sweepstake about the arrival date of your baby. Ask people at work, in the pub, or relatives and friends to guess the baby's birthday. Give them the doctor's estimated date and let them have a little flutter. Of course, you'll have the inside information so you'll be odds-on favourite to win. But don't let that stop you having a bet yourself.

Val: 'We sold sweepstake tickets throughout my office for 50p each. The prize money was enough to keep a Fleet Street boozer afloat for days. But guess who the lucky winner was? Me and the doctor who helped me to succeed with a mere minute to spare.'

2   Photograph yourself in all your bulging beauty. You may never look this way again so why not keep a pictorial record? Even better, have your man click the shutter while you pose tastefully in the nude or near-nude. For a top model result take off all your underwear an hour before the photo session so that the elastic marks of your bra and knickers will fade away. Rub some oil on your shoulders, breasts and tummy for a soft, dewy look, and don't slouch. Make sure you sit up straight, and remember that a side view is more flattering than a full front. It also shows off your beautiful bulge much better.

3   Spoil yourself somehow. If there is anything that never fails to make you feel sensational this is the time to have it. Whether it's a facial, new make-up, or a gallon of ex-

pensive scent, a movie-star-style bubble bath or eating peanut butter sandwiches in bed for a whole day, you need it. We know a girl who woke up at 1.00 a.m. and said: 'I'm going to have a baby soon so I think I deserve a picnic – now!' Luckily she had a well-stocked fridge and an understanding bloke!

4 Get a wash-and-wear hairstyle. Find the best hair stylist in your area and get a really easy-to-care for cut. Once you become a mother you won't have much time for pincurls, heated rollers or elaborate topknots. Not at first, anyway. So you need a hairstyle which will survive the labour ward and still look presentable while you're in hospital. A really ritzy hairdo is not an extravagance under these circumstances. And it's a great morale-booster. (Don't have a perm because pregnancy sometimes badly affects the hair and perms don't 'take'.)

5 Glamour dates. In Australia some mother-loving genius dreamed up the idea of maternity hospitals babysitting on the last night of a new mother's stay. This allows her and her husband to have a last night out together without any worries about their baby. These hospitals realise it may be months before couples have the opportunity to step out again. Mothers in this country have no such luck. So now is the time to catch the film or show you've been longing to see, try that new exotic restaurant or go to a rock concert.

6 Buy a nearly-nightie. You won't believe it but you will feel sexy and seductive again one day. And you will be slim again, you will! Choosing a wisp of a nightgown for that apparently far-distant day is another great way to boost your morale. Pack it away in a scented drawer until you get home from hospital.

Soothing the Savage Beast Inside your Man

One of the last but most important things you must do before you go to hospital is stock up your larder. What's going to keep your man alive in your absence? Okay, it *should* be the least of your problems. Any man who can't boil an egg or open a can deserves to starve. But it's as well to remember that new dads are too excited and busy rushing from hospital to home, fetching, carrying and doing your hospital laundry, to shop or cook for themselves. And in-between all this scurrying around they're expected to go to work, too. (An excellent reason paternity leave should be given to all new fathers by law.)

Both our blokes underwent personality changes when they became new dads. They suffered from too much wetting the babies' heads. And too much rushing from work for hospital visiting hours – to say nothing of the night's sleep they lost helping us through long labours. (Both our babies arrived in the early hours of the morning.)

On the great day when we brought our babies home from the hospital we had two exhausted, ravenously hungry men.

Val: 'I cooked a Shepherds Pie for 6, planning to put half in the freezer in preparation for a tough few weeks ahead. Before the pie reached the table my husband scoffed the lot, then said: "Get your hands out of the way, otherwise I'll eat them, too".'

Judy: 'As soon as I arrived home the baby went to bed in her new crib. And when I looked around her dad had keeled over and gone to sleep too. I found him crashed out, fully dressed, and he didn't stir until the next morning. Not surprising since he'd been too excited to sleep the previous 4 nights. At least he was more comfortable collapsed in his clothes than in a train at the end of the line – which is where he woke one day at 3.00 a.m. after sleeping through his stop.'

Even a freezerful of meals-for-one won't tempt a really tired new father. So if you can't call on a neighbour or relative to shove a hot dinner through the letterbox to the hungry beast inside your house, leave the phone numbers and addresses of your nearest fast-food cafes. Take away meals now come in many varieties ranging from Chinese and Indian to British-style chicken and chips.

And leave some goodies to nibble in the kitchen cupboards as well as some tins of his favourite canned foods with an opener nearby. This is NOT pampering your man. Call it a bit of insurance. A happy homecoming may be spoiled if you have a starving, worn out man around the house. After all, you want him to take more interest in his new family than in his food, don't you?

Minor Hassles of Late Pregnancy

As if you didn't have enough to worry about now, this stage often brings a few extra irritations. None of these is serious, just annoying.

Cramps in legs and feet

Cause: some doctors blame calcium deficiency in the body. Solution: persuade your fella to massage the cramped muscles vigorously with baby lotion for several minutes. Putting a pillow under the bottom of the mattress on your side of the bed so that your feet are raised all night also helps. Try wiggling your foot upwards, downwards and in circles while you clasp your ankle to help the motion. A bedtime drink of milk may help to put more calcium into your system. And an old wives' tale which, we're told, really works is to put a magnet under the bedclothes.

Shortness of breath

Cause: enlarged uterus pushing the stomach up under the ribs and diaphragm. Difficult to take deep breaths. Solution: don't lie flat. Prop yourself up on a couple of pillows. The problem disappears after the 'lightening', when the baby's head drops into the pelvic area about four weeks before the birth.

Swelling (Oedema)

Cause: you're sloshing around with about 10 pints of fluid in your tissues during the last 2 months. So your legs, ankles and face may become very swollen. Unimportant when it happens at the end of the day, but if your legs swell early in the day this may be a warning of toxaemia. See your doctor at once. Solution: keep your feet up as much as possible. Watch your weight. Overweight women tend to suffer more with this condition.

Bleeding gums and nose

Cause: increased blood supply surging through your system. This is a very common side-effect. Solution: for bleeding gums see your dentist. You may need a softer toothbrush. Nose bleeds: just pinch and press nasal passages together. Don't tip your head backwards. If your nasal tissues are dry and likely to crack rub petroleum jelly into each nostril.

Backache

Cause: strain on the lower spine. Result of extra weight in pregnancy. Aggravated by bad posture of too much weight gain. Solution: best cure is prevention. Good posture essential. Lots of rest. Wear shoes of the same heel height all the time. Massage and hot water bottle pressed against back may help.

Stomach pains

Cause: stretching of ligaments supporting the womb. Usually more painful on right side than left. Doesn't do any harm. Doesn't need treatment. Will disappear around 32nd week. Solution: rest.

Tail pain

Cause: overweight and bad posture – lounging or slouch-
ing. Makes sitting for long periods painful. Solution:
massage, better posture and weight watching. Walk tall
with stomach and tail tucked in, shoulders back.

Heartburn

Cause: hormone which softens a valve at top of the
stomach. Some acid from stomach gets into food pipe.
Produces searing pain in lower chest. But not connected
with heart. Solution: avoid spicy foods. Try milk of mag-
nesia or even small glass of milk. This counteracts acidity
in stomach.

Varicose veins

Cause: constant extra pressure on the veins. Solution: no
real solution. but watch your weight. Avoid standing for
long stretches. May be hereditary. More likely to occur in
second or subsequent pregnancies. Never wear tight
elasticised underwear or girdles. Use a footstool when
sitting. Never cross your legs as this obstructs blood flow.
Use support hose to prevent veins getting worse.

Piles

Cause: straining as a result of constipation. Solution:
avoid this by eating more roughage in your diet; wholewheat brown bread, muesli, fresh fruit and vegetables all
help. Ask your doctor for a special ointment which relieves
pain and swelling.

Constipation

Cause: sometimes the hormone progesterone softens the
intestine and prevents the bowels from working effectively.

Iron tablets prescribed for pregnancy may aggravate this condition. Solution: as well as roughage suggested above, drink a minimum of 4 pints of fluid a day.

Insomnia

Cause: unusually vigorous movements of baby in the middle of night. Also, extreme body temperatures either very hot or cold. Solution: warm or cool drinks, warm bath. If desire to pee wakes you up avoid drinks 2 hours before bedtime. Otherwise try listening to the radio or reading a dull book once you wake. And catch up on your sleep by catnapping during the day. If insomnia becomes serious problem consult your doctor.

Ante-natal depression:

Cause: natural fears about the birth. Or sometimes a woman who gives up her job too soon sits at home and feels miserable. Solution: work out the cause. Discuss it with your man or any sympathetic friend. Try any of the daffy ideas we suggested for jazzing up your last dreary weeks on page 108).

Crazy Cravings

Cause: as yet unknown. Many women have a yen for sharp acid tastes like pickles. Or weird combinations like ice cream and chutney. Solution: these fads and fancies shouldn't worry you. They don't harm the baby and usually vanish as quickly as they came. Indulge them a little if you must.

Absentmindedness

Cause: unknown. But can be embarrassing.

Val: 'I went to the dentist and saw him looking down

at my feet. Eventually, he said: "I like your right shoe much more than the left". I looked down and saw not only two entirely different shoes, but also a difference of two inches in the heel heights. I'd been hobbling around all day thinking the baby was lying more on my right side than my left.'

Solution: make lists of things you mustn't forget. And always check your appeareance in a mirror before you leave home.

CHAPTER TEN

How To Be Hip in Hospital

After 9 months of waiting your baby is finally on her way into the world. So you grab your suitcase and head for the hospital when one or more signs of labour has appeared. (*See* Chapter 11.)

When you arrive at the hospital you'll be feeling excited and probably nervous, expecially if this is your first baby. But the orderly routine of the hospital has a curiously calming effect. A nurse will take your case and accompany you to the labour ward where you'll be examined by a doctor or midwife. He (or she) will take your temperature, blood pressure and listen to the baby's heart just like a routine examination at your ante-natal clinic.

After you are tucked up in bed a nurse will ask you to sign a consent form. This is a legal document which states that in the event of any emergency, medical staff may carry out any procedure they think necessary. Unless you sign it you may be refused treatment.

Friend or Enema?

Not long after you've settled into bed you'll be offered the twin terrors of British maternity hospitals: an enema and shaving off your pubic hair. Both are more undignified than uncomfortable, but many people believe, as we do, that they are also unnecessary today.

An enema is used to empty your bowels at the start of labour so that no accidental mess will mar the delivery. This would embarrass the mother and create extra work for the nurses. But having an enema is not exactly a fun time. A thin rubber hose is gently pushed into your back passage and warm soapy water is poured down it.

This doesn't hurt, but most of us are not used to long rubber hoses disappearing into such places, so may tense up and make the job more difficult. The trick is to relax your bottom, lie back and think of the person you'd most like to have an enema. Maybe this isn't Christian but it makes you feel a lot better!

An enema takes effect almost instantly which can mean a frantic dash for the nearest lavatory. The whole process is even more uncomfortable when you're dealing with contractions at the same time.

Are enemas really necessary? Suppositories, which are long pellets containing laxatives, do the same job if a little more slowly. They are much easier to insert and kinder to your bottom. In fact, lots of hospitals now prefer them. But some still insist that only an enema works thoroughly. We feel it's worth asking for a suppository if you have a choice.

Full Frontal Defuzzing

In the bad old days you lost your pubic hair along with your dignity because doctors believed shaving prevented infection. Recent research shows that infections are slightly less likely if pubic hair stays put. Now some of the more modern hospitals limit shaving to the area immediately around the birth canal. This is absolutely painless and takes around four seconds to complete.

The reason for still doing this quick lather-and-scrape? Just in case you have an episiotomy (a cut at the outlet of the birth canal to make your delivery easier). If this area is clean of hair the stitches used to sew up the cut won't be tangled with hair. And if you've ever been caught by the 'short-and-curlies' you'll know the nurse who wields the razor is doing you a favour!

If hospital staff want to give you a full frontal defuzzing and whisk off every single hair we think you should protest loudly. It's just not necessary.

Tips to make you a Star Patient

Hospital staff are usually busy and often overworked. So how do you make them feel your case is special when what's thrilling to you is routine for them? Here are some tips that may help:

1 Don't drive staff crazy with unnecessary demands for attention. If you have the father or a close friend beside you he can give you all the small personal attentions that hospital staff are just too busy to do. Like fetching drinks of water, wiping your forehead, rubbing your back and reading to you.

2 Most mums are keen to know how they are progressing but are either too shy to ask questions, or too zonked out by drugs to take an interest. By being in control of your labour you can remain alert and involved to the end. This means you can ask sensible questions, such as how far the cervix is dilated. (For a baby to pass into the birth canal your cervix should be widened from a pencil-thin slit to ten centimetres.)

3 Remember the little courtesies, if you can. A mother who is not doped up with painkillers can say 'please' and 'thank you'; and everyone loves being treated politely. Some women get completely out of control when they strike the rough patches in labour. They scream and swear at everyone in earshot. Although the nurses won't enjoy your performance they'll be more understanding if your previous behaviour has shown them you're not a fulltime bitch. (But faithfully following your breathing exercises in labour should make the rougher sections easier to handle.)

4 If you want hospital staff to take an interest in you,

show some interest in *them*. Many nurses and doctors come from abroad. In the first stage of labour when contractions are light you could ask a few friendly questions about their homelands – even if you make a gaffe and discover that kind nurse with a foreign name was born right here in Britain.

A nutty beauty we know decided that the most vital part of producing a baby was getting some superb needlework in the vagina when the doctor stitched up her episiotomy after the birth. Unfortunately, it was 3.00 a.m. when her baby arrived and a woman doctor had to be called from a sound sleep to sew her up. Although our friend wasn't feeling very chatty she switched on all the high-powered charm she could muster. The result was after a long, careful sewing job the doctor looked up and said: 'I'm really proud of my work. I have repaired you so beautifully your husband will come back and thank me in a few week's time.'

5   If you have brightened up your pregnancy by running a sweepstake on the baby's arrival date now is the time this may pay unexpected dividends.

Val: 'It was almost 11.30 p.m. on the day I bet my baby would arrive before midnight. So I told the doctor on duty all about the vast sums that were within my reach. He laughed and said he'd do his best to make my child arrive a rich kid. My daughter was born at a minute to midnight. I'm sure he didn't speed up the birth unnecessarily to help me win, but the fun sweepstake helped to cheer both of us while we worked. Later, I sent him a bottle of good wine and a thank you note describing the wine's aphrodisiac qualities.'

CHAPTER ELEVEN

Birth Rights and Wrongs

If you could have your second baby first this chapter might not be necessary. Usually only the actual experience of giving birth can tell you which type of delivery suits you best. Many women have unhappy experiences during childbirth because they're not fully prepared and don't know what to expect. So they have treatments they don't understand or want.

For more than 100 years childbirth has been controlled by doctors, usually male. And no man, however well-meaning or sensitive, can understand what giving birth really feels like. The result is that women today are not in charge of the most important event in their lives.

Birth has become more mechanised, something done to you rather than something you take pride in doing yourself. The medical team, their machines and instruments now bring the baby into the world instead of a mother's natural efforts.

But research is beginning to show that unhappy experiences during childbirth can seriously affect a woman's feelings about motherhood for months and even years afterwards. Dr. Sam Baxter of London's Charing Cross Hospital says: 'You can't expect women to enjoy birth when hospitals treat pregnancy as a disease. It's a conveyor-belt, alien system treating people just like robots. What a woman needs is a positive atmosphere in which to give birth to become a normal, responsive mother afterwards.' He also thinks that the problem of frigidity which many women experience after childbirth could be connected with their treatment in hospital.

Medical writer Dr. Oliver Gillie goes even further: 'For the world around it (childbirth) is commonplace – just another baby. Parents often have to argue to have their special needs and interests understood. Expert though the maternity services are in saving life, their understanding of emotional needs has too often been dismal.'[1]

But expectant parents can do a great deal to make sure their baby is born the way they choose. Before deciding which kind of childbirth you want, find out about your local hospital. Either ask your doctor about the methods used there or visit the maternity unit to see for yourself.

Then when you have the information you need, ask yourself what matters most to you. For instance, do you want a labour which begins naturally? Or would you be grateful if your doctor suggested an induction to start labour and get it over quickly? Would you like a natural childbirth relying on special breathing exercises to relieve birth pangs? Or would you prefer the newest painkilling drugs? How strongly do you feel about having your baby beside you throughout the day and night in hospital? Would you be happier if your baby disappeared into a nursery so you could rest?

Most hospitals don't offer patients much choice, but it's always worth asking for what you want. The newer the hospital the more likely you are to find staff more receptive to pleasing the patient.

How to Get What You Want

When you've made your choice ask your doctor to help you get what you want. It's always best to have him (or her) on your side. If he can't, or won't help, write to your Regional Hospital Board. (Get the address from your town hall or library.) Ask the Board for a list of hospitals in your area using the methods you prefer to deliver babies. When you get this list write to the Secretary of the hospital of your choice.

In your letter state clearly which treatments you do or do not want. For example, if you ever felt claustrophobic having a gas and air mask at the dentist you may be upset by having this during labour. So make certain you mention this reason in your letter.

To be fair you should add: '*Naturally, I will consent to all necessary procedures taken in an emergency. I simply wish such procedures to be explained to me.*' When the hospital answers your letter you'll then have written proof that it agrees to all or some of your requests. If you're satisfied with this reply ask your doctor to book you in. Bear in mind that if the hospital goes against your expressed wishes you may have grounds for sueing it.

If possible, ask your man to sign this letter too. It's one more way of involving him in the birth. And his signature may help should your letter end up on the desk of a fuddy-duddy male who dislikes anything that's not routine, especially if suggested by a woman. And there are more of this type still around than you'd like to think! The only snag in this lovely scheme may be that you have only one hospital in your area, so no choice at all. If this is the case then try to get a consultant gynaecologist in charge of your case who is sympathetic to your idea. (Often two or more consultants work at the same hospital.)

All this hassle may seem boring and needless but remember it's not only for your benefit, but designed to give your baby a happy entry into this world. Thousands of women complain each year that their baby's birth was spoiled because they were given treatments in labour which they didn't want and didn't like. And recent research shows that an anxious unhappy mother is more likely to produce a distressed baby. So all this ground work is a kind of insurance policy to ensure your baby's birth will be something you'll remember afterwards with pleasure.

Your Choice of Pain Relievers

Painless childbirth is experienced only by a lucky few. Most of us need some kind of help to cope with contractions especially in the tougher, late stages of labour. For some women controlled breathing may be all they need. Other, perhaps older women whose muscle tone is not so supple may need extra help. Fortunately for them modern science has found various ways to assist almost everyone to have an easier time.

These painkillers do relieve birth pangs in varying degrees but they have one disadvantage. All of them may get into your baby's system by crossing over the placenta. And a normal dose for a grown woman may be an overdose for a tiny baby. The danger is that they may drug the baby and depress her ability to breathe and suckle. Dr. Charles Richard Gilbert, a leading American obstetrician says: 'The perfect analgesic or anaesthetic has not been discovered. All have drawbacks.'[2] And British obstetrician Geoffrey Chamberlain says: 'No drug can be said to be absolutely blame-free.' He suggests patients say to their doctors: 'Just in case this drug has an effect on my baby that you don't know about yet, I won't take it.'[3]

We feel that there is not yet sufficient research on the long-term effects of most of these pain killers. So natural childbirth, using controlled breathing, still seems to us the safest possible way to have your baby. And if you do need a little extra help towards the end of your labour at least you won't have relied on painkillers totally, and you will have reduced the possible ill-effects on your baby to the minimum.

Here are the pain relievers generally available in Britain together with their advantages and known disadvantages:

1 *Controlled Breathing:* The natural childbirth method using special breathing exercises can be very effective if you keep concentrating and stay in the rhythm of it. This works by preparing you for the whole process of giving birth. You learn the correct way to breathe so you can relax all the muscles in your body and avoid tensing up which blocks the baby's struggles to be born, thereby causing the worst pain. Controlled breathing teaches you to co-operate with the baby's and your body. The exercises you learn are not

difficult and really work, but they're also monotonous.
Concentrating may be difficult in a busy labour ward. But we
still feel this is the best way to go through labour because
your own efforts actually help your baby. So you have a
marvellous feeling of accomplishment. (*See* page 85.)

2 *Injected Painkillers:* Pethidine: an injection usually in the
rump to reduce the painful effect of contractions. Takes
about 10–15 minutes before you get any noticeable relief and
lasts roughly 4 hours. You may feel fine, even a bit tiddly
and therefore unable to concentrate on your breathing exercises. Doctors are now becoming concerned about the effect
of pethidine on the newborn. A study at the University
Hospital of Wales in Cardiff revealed depressed breathing in
babies whose mothers had pethidine injections.

3 *Epidural Anaesthesia:* An injection in the spinal cord which
relieves pain totally in over 90 per cent of women. Numbs the
entire birth area from belly down to toes. All normal birth
sensations are deadened. Kills the urge to push and therefore
usually results in a forceps delivery (which usually means
the father will not be allowed to see the delivery). Not
generally available yet but gaining popularity. Effects on
the mother may be a drop in blood pressure, nausea and
vomiting. Effects on the baby may include limp muscles, and
a decreased rooting activity (less able to find mother's
breast).

Val: 'After 8 hours in labour I was coping beautifully
        with my breathing exercises when several doctors
        offered me an epidural. They warned that my
        labour would be long and that I'd be much too
        tired to push the baby out, so I gave in. In fact,
        the delivery wasn't difficult and if I'd known this,
        I'd never have agreed to an epidural. Perhaps
        hospitals are so pleased with their new gadgets
        they're too keen to see patients using them.
        Though painfree, (you can't feel even a twinge)

an epidural is scarey because you can't feel your
legs or move them. After my baby was born one
of my legs slipped off the bed. A nurse had to
lift it back on, I couldn't! One girl in my ward
said she'd slept through all her contractions and
had to be woken up to give birth. Not the most
memorable way to have a baby.'

4 *Paracervical Block:* A local anaesthetic, only used in the first
stage of labour when the cervix is dilated less than five centimetres. Brings total pain relief for up to 4 hours in most cases.
Not as popular in Britain as in America and Scandinavia
where it is widely used.

5 *Pudendal Nerve Block:* Usually used only with a forceps
delivery. When the baby's head is about to appear and the
tissues around the vagina are very stretched you may feel
you're going to rip. This local injection cuts out any discomfort. Takes effect at once. But you lose the sensation of
the baby rushing out from the birth canal.

6 *Acupuncture:* You can have your baby the pins and needles
way with this ancient form of pain relief from Asia. It's just
beginning to be accepted in the West.

Judy: 'I was only the second mother in Britain to have
my baby with acupuncture. Thanks to the
gynaecologist in my NHS hospital who was
interested in seeing it work, I managed to find
a reliable acupuncturist through the Acupuncture
Association (*see* page 263 for their address).

'My labour was induced with just a few needles
stuck between two toes on both feet and a few
around my knees. It sounds barbaric but I
couldn't feel them going in and in fact, had a
beautiful floating feeling. I couldn't feel any
contractions once they started. But the hospital
staff could, when they touched my belly. The
only trouble was that, as the hours wore on, I
found it increasingly difficult to lie still. I was

warned if I moved I might dislodge the needles so I began to get very stiff and as the contractions began to get stronger I started to feel them. I got other aches and pains as my muscles stiffened. Finally when the contractions were really intense, I found that my breathing exercises were just as helpful as the acupuncture. I was also *very* grateful for the gas-and-air mask offered by a nurse. So acupuncture was not a total success for me. The acupuncturist said I wasn't an ideal subject because I was super-sensitive to pain, but I felt that my labour might have been shorter and more comfortable if I had been able to turn and move about and so keep my muscles more supple.'

7 *Hypnosis:* This seems to be a much more successful way of avoiding pain in childbirth – if you're the type who makes a good subject for hypnosis. Over 2,000 babies have been delivered this way in Britain. Mrs. Susan Simpson who had her baby by hypnosis in the London Hospital, Mile End says: 'I'd say I felt about 20 per cent of the pain normally associated with labour. When 80 per cent flies out of the window, you're lucky.'[4]

Hypnosis works like this: a hypnotist helps you to relax and calm down, then repeats certain soothing phrases: 'You're feeling drowsy, drowsy and comfy, your eyes are closing . . . etc.' Eventually a mother learns to hypnotise herself to feel excitement and pleasure, not fear or pain. The advantage of this method is that you are fully conscious and can actively help your baby to be born without pain.

If you'd like to try this method, ask your G.P. if any facilities operate in your area.

Your Choice of Childbirth

1 *Induction:* A controversial method of artificially starting and speeding up labour. The bag of waters around the baby

is ruptured (usually with a blunt instrument) and a hormone drip (usually Oxytocin or Syntocinon) is inserted in a vein in your hand. The hormone stimulates the muscles of the uterus to push the baby out. New research indicates that rupturing the bag of waters is not a good idea. This bag cushions the infant's head against the powerful battering it receives while passing through the mother's cervix and pelvic floor. Without its protective buffer the baby could suffer a disalignment of the skullbones which now occurs twice as often as in babies born spontaneously.

Doctors say induction makes births safer to explain why figures for induced births have nearly trebled in 10 years. Surely the risks to babies at birth haven't trebled in the same time? Only between 10 and 15 per cent of all births in Britain are likely to develop complications and these will mostly be minor ones. For this unlucky few induced births may be necessary. But the pioneer of induced births in the U.K., Dr. Alex Turnbull, Nuffield Professor of Gynaecology at Oxford University says: 'A real analysis of the situation now suggests that the technique is not as good as we thought it would be.'[5] Nearly a quarter (22.4 per cent) of speeded up babies show some distress after birth compared with only 13.5 per cent of other babies. And 4 times as many induced babies need special care at birth.

Contractions are also far more intense after you've been induced. One young mum's experience: 'I'd gone to relaxation classes but found that I was totally unprepared for the different type of pain I experienced. I thought labour would go in stages. With induction, the contractions did not build up slowly as they normally do but were terrifically strong right from the start. The result was that I couldn't get into the rhythym of the breathing exercises, couldn't use them therefore, so had a far more difficult labour. I'm determined not to be induced for my next child, unless there's a really good medical reason for it.'

Induction is *usually* not necessary just because your baby is a week or two overdue. Also, if you're not sure about the date of your last period, you could induce a baby prematurely.

So make sure of the reason if your doctor suggests induction. If you're uncertain, it's quite in order to ask for another opinion. Only agree if you understand their reasons. (*Also see* page 130).

2 *Normal Delivery.* (Spontaneous Vaginal Delivery): Most babies are born head first, face down. Then the head rotates to one side as it slides out. No artifical help, like forceps, is necessary.

3 *Premature Labour :* If your baby arrives four or more weeks before her expected date, and weighs less than 5 lbs, she's called premature. Very much smaller premature babies have survived – a celebrated case was a boy weighing 1 lb. 12 ozs. who survived. No one knows the exact reason for labour beginning early but many doctors suspect one cause could be toxaemia.

4 *Breech Birth :* The baby is born the wrong way round, emerging bottom first. This usually means a more compli-cated labour, therefore it must take place in hospital. One in every 20 births is a breech delivery.

5 *Forceps Delivery :* Sometimes, a baby needs extra help to be born. So metal instruments called forceps gently clamp around the baby's head and she's slowly pulled out. This might result in some bruising of your vaginal area. The baby's head could show bruising marks, as well.

6 *Caesarian Birth :* Named after Julius Caesar who was born by this method. Used if the mother's pelvic bones are too small for the size of the baby's head or if there is some risk to the baby in an over-long labour. Surgery is used to remove the baby from the womb. The mother has a general or epidural anaesthetic and sometimes doesn't have any birth pangs.

The Right Questions at the Right Time

To remain the star of your show throughout labour you need all your wits about you. This is a time when you probably feel very vulnerable. The clinical and unfamiliar surroundings of hospital make you feel a little lost. And the starched, white uniform of the staff could intimidate anyone. Uniforms lend people an air of authority and some of us feel that we must agree with whatever the medical staff suggest.

Despite all this you can keep in touch with what's happening to you and control your own labour. Try not to feel nervous. Ask the medical team intelligent questions at the right moment. Having your man or a friend to speak up for you can often make all the difference.

Nurses and midwives will pop into your room and do mysterious things like peering at your innards and writing mystifying marks on charts. They'll be in a rush but if you ask they'll explain all these procedures. And it's reassuring to know everything is going smoothly. This is yet another reason for you to stay alert, and on top of your labour – which means not relying on drugs too much.

Some of the questions you may want to ask could include these:

1 The doctor suggests that the birth be induced. You ask politely: 'Could you please explain why you think this is necessary?' If his explanation satisfies you, agree. If not ask more questions until you *are* satisfied. One of our friends agreed to be induced a week early. She found out afterwards that the real reason for this was the baby's scheduled arrival date clashed with the doctor's holiday plans! If you are not satisfied with any explanation the doctor gives and you are against induction in principle ask for a second opinion from another doctor.

2 When a nurse measures how far your cervix has opened up ask her: 'Can you please tell me how wide it is now?' When she tells you ask her to guess when you'll deliver.

It's amazing how a possible time limit can keep you going.

3 If you're against the idea of an episiotomy make sure the midwife or doctor knows how strongly you feel. Get your man to tell the delivery team too. If they insist ask: 'Please let me push a little longer.' If you find 10 minutes or so extra pushing doesn't work, it's reasonable to give in. (*See* page 140.)

4 Some questions may be less important medically but concern matters which may boost your morale – like make-up. You may find a bossy sister dead against patients wearing powder or mascara in a labour ward. A crazy redhead we know had an argument between contractions with a starchy nurse who wanted her red toe-nail polish to come off. Surely a little nail polish couldn't endanger a baby?

Val: 'I wore "permanent" false eyelashes during my delivery and looked gorgeous, I thought. Until the lashes wilted along with the rest of me after many hours in labour.'

CHAPTER TWELVE

Happy Birth Day

Labour often begins just like a love affair – you wonder if this time it's the real thing. Sometimes women who aren't sure dash off to hospital only to be sent straight home again. But the earliest and surest warning that your baby is getting ready to appear comes a few weeks before the birth. That's when the baby's head moves down into the pelvis. Sometimes this is called 'lightening'. Your doctor will tell you that the head is now 'engaged', which means in position ready to be born. With the baby lower the pressure against your lungs and diaphragm is reduced so you may find you can breathe more easily.

Many expectant mums have at least one false alarm. But when the baby is really on her way you will have one of three clear signs – a show, or contractions, or breaking of the waters.

1 *The Show :* When you go to the lavatory you'll notice streaks of pinky blood mixed sometimes with a lump of clear jellied mucous. Like a stopper in the neck of a bottle this plugs up the cervix or neck of the womb to prevent any infection reaching the baby inside. When the cervix begins stretching as labour starts a small amount of blood may escape to give you this early warning sign. But if you notice a lot of blood, enough to soak a sanitary pad, you should contact your doctor at once.

2 *Contractions :* A contraction is the tensing and relaxing of muscles. And the womb is made up of groups of muscles. During labour these clench and unclench to move the baby

downwards into the birth canal. Right throughout pregnancy your womb is contracting at intervals of about 15 minutes, but generally you aren't aware of this. From about the 36th week you may get weak contractions lasting about 30 seconds. These soften and prepare the cervix to let the baby through. They are called Braxton Hicks contractions after the man who first noted them.

What contractions feel like: At first labour contractions are short and weak, lasting about 20 to 30 seconds. You'll probably feel only a slight stiffness across your belly as the womb tightens up in first stage labour. Gradually they build up becoming stronger and longer until by the end of the first stage they each last about 90 seconds. The feeling is rather like period pains (although much more powerful) because the contractions come in waves rising and flowing away across the lower stomach. Just like a wide belt around your abdomen a contraction gets tighter, tighter and tighter. Then slowly the 'belt' loosens until the feeling is completely gone.

These sensations are more strenuous than painful. The feeling is not the same as the ache from a broken limb or surgery. It's a positive, creative kind of pain because each contraction is bringing you closer to your goal. You can comfort yourself after each one knowing you have one less to cope with.

Two extreme views of contractions:

'I can only describe what I felt as something like butterflies in the tummy. There was no pain or real discomfort at all. The baby arrived two hours after I arrived at the hospital. And the staff just wouldn't believe it was my first. I heard one of the nurses say: "She must be fibbing". If I had the strength I'd have got up and sloshed her one. But then the baby shot out so fast it almost hit the opposite wall.'

Dancer, aged 25.

'I spent the night before my baby was induced in a ward next to the delivery room. I couldn't sleep because women giving birth in the next room were screaming their heads off all night. They sounded as if they were having their toenails ripped off or somethin'. Instead of being frightened by their screams I just thought to meself: "Silly cows! I won't make a big fuss like that". But those ladies were quiet compared with me when I got going. My husband said they could hear me on the other side of town.'

Lancashire mother of two.

3 *The waters break:* Your baby is swimming in a bag of amniotic fluid which often bursts and drains away at the beginning of labour. If this happens line your knickers with a sanitary pad and contact your hospital immediately. They will probably ask you to come straight in.

During the last weeks of pregnancy many women are worried that they'll go shopping one day and flood the supermarket. But it rarely happens like this. And if the baby's head is engaged in the pelvis the water is blocked off and can't escape. But it's a good idea to put a rubber waterproof sheet or several old towels on your bed to protect your mattress while you sleep. Of course, accidents in public can happen, although they are comparatively rare. A famous British actress couldn't resist catching a big opening night of a play even though her third baby was due the same day. In the middle of the exciting last act her waters broke. 'I did so want to see the end,' she said later, 'so I just waited till the curtain fell then splashed my way out and went to hospital.'

As each of these symptoms appears look at your watch and write down the time on a piece of paper which you can take to the hospital. They'll add this information to your case notes.

Usually labour starts with contractions. Frequently these begin in the middle of the night because you are warm, comfortable and relaxed. So don't jump out of bed and begin bustling around getting ready. If you do, chances are the contractions will go away again. As contractions come just relax, give in to them and start your breathing exercises. In this way the rest of your body is not using up energy that the womb could use to get on with its job.

Remember, and this goes for the whole of your labour, the minute you tighten your muscles and fight contractions rather than giving in to them, you will experience pain. If you co-operate, relax and let go with each contraction, the discomfort will be greatly reduced.

Get up slowly at your usual time and have a warm bath. This isn't to make you clean. The warm water will stimulate the blood to your tummy and make the abdominal contractions easier to deal with.

Have a light breakfast such as a boiled egg with toast. Make sure your fella has a decent breakfast too. If he's going with you to the hospital it may be a long time before he gets another good meal. A light breakfast will give you a reserve of energy which will help you at the start of labour. If you don't eat now you'll become tired and weak sooner and probably have a more difficult time. In mid-labour your digestive system closes down while your body concentrates all its efforts on the birth so you won't be allowed food at that stage.

Try to do everything in a calm, unhurried way so you don't waste any energy. You'll need every bit for the tough job ahead. (After all, labour gets its name because it means hard work.) It's probably the hardest job you'll ever do in your life. So every time you have a contraction flop into a chair and give in to it by controlling your breathing. The longer you carry on like this in your own familiar surroundings the better. Doctors say the most common mistake in labour is to rush to the hospital too soon. But when a contraction lasts for about 60 seconds you'll know your labour is well established and you should then leave for the hospital.

First Stage Labour

This is the longest, most boring and usually most uncomfortable stretch of labour. No one can tell accurately how long it will last. This depends on the time it takes for your cervix to widen. In a first birth this may be 12 hours or more. A second is usually much quicker.

After your contractions, pulse, blood pressure and everything else have been checked in the labour ward, the nurses will give you and your man some peace and quiet, 'to get on with it'. At this stage, all you can do is wait as the contractions grow stronger and the cervix widens. While you wait, here are four tips to make labour more interesting and less draggy:

1 At regular intervals throughout labour, a nurse will listen to your baby's heartbeat. To give you a bit of a boost, why not ask the nurse to let you listen, too? Some foetal heart monitors have an amplifier so that the whole room is flooded with the healthy throb of your unborn child's heart.

2 Guess your baby's sex by timing those heartbeats. A well-known London gynaecologist has a 100 per cent success rate foretelling the sex of her patients' babies. She believes boys have a slower heart rate – around 120 beats per minute; while girls' hearts beat faster – about 140–160 beats per minute. All we can say about this is that it worked for us and a lot of our friends.

3 You'll find that music may help to take your mind off your surroundings. Why not ask your fella (or whoever is with you) to bring a transistor radio or portable tape recorder. Have your contractions to the beat of a rumba or rock 'n' roll. (Time your breathing to the strong rhythm of the music as well.) Playing music softly shouldn't disturb anyone, and you can turn it off when a doctor or midwife examines you. It could soothe not only you and your husband but your baby as well! (If you can, persuade the nurse to dim the lights a little, while you wait. It may be more difficult to arrange but it's worth trying.)

4 Your husband can make the birth even more memorable by recording the whole process on film or on tape.

Hospitals usually permit this if you ask in advance – though there are limits. A London teaching hospital drew the line when one proud dad – a professional film maker – turned up with several cameras, tripods, umbrella reflectors and a sound recordist in tow!

It's in this early waiting stage that you'll really appreciate the company of your man or a close friend. He can make himself useful mopping your brow, giving you sips of water, massaging your aching back or just holding your hand. At the height of a contraction, he can help to take your mind off the pain in your belly by squeezing your wrist tightly. And he can fend off well-meaning questions from the nursing staff such as 'How are we coming along now?' by explaining that you can't answer right now because you're busy handling a contraction.

Medical staff have set ideas about how a woman should spend labour. You're expected to lie down on a high bed either on your back or your side. But western women appear to be the only ones who go through labour like this. Medical writer Oliver Gillie says: 'In most other cultures women kneel, squat, crouch or sit. When a woman lies on her back the weight of the baby and womb rests on major blood vessels underneath preventing blood from circulating normally.' He adds: 'When a woman is lying on her back she has to push a baby uphill and the area around the birth canal is then tighter and may stretch less easily.'[1]

Doctors in Scandinavia and America have found that delivery is easier and quicker if a woman sits up. In this way she avoids the intense back pain caused by lying in one position for hours, which many women experience during labour. A sitting position also means gravity is helping to deliver the baby, so it drops down into the birth canal faster.

Giving birth this way is one more centuries-old idea which is now gaining favour with progressive obstetricians. And many so-called primitive aids to childbirth now seem worth reconsidering.

Labour is a very basic function and, according to the

National Childbirth Trust, it's been found that a woman's psychological needs become basic, too. One of the needs a woman returns to is the urge to suck. They suggest soaking a small sponge in water and sucking this as your mouth gets very dry during labour.[2] The sponge could also come in useful to wipe over the lower part of your face and neck. (Your man should change the water for the sponge often.)

He should also remind you to empty your bladder every hour. You'll need a reminder because you may lose the urge to pee when the baby's head presses downwards. And a full bladder slows down the opening of the cervix and makes labour more painful. If your bladder is emptied regularly you won't need to have a catheter inserted to drain it artificially.

Reducing Fear

In this first stage you may feel scared because you have weird sensations in your body which you can't control. Dr. Rosamond Bischoff thinks this fear is transmitted to the baby who becomes frightened, too. She suggests one way to help the baby and yourself at the same time is to talk to her. Put your hand over your belly and tell her quietly or even silently that everything is all right – you're both working together and you'll be fine. Dr. Bischoff says: 'You'll be surprised at the way your body will react. Muscles, nerves, womb will often relax more if the mother is in this constructive frame of mind. I've known colleagues to scoff at this until they've actually seen it happen. Your comforting message gets through to the baby through nerve endings and blood vessels. 'Many labour wards actually physically smell of fear from women who are not properly prepared for birth. The fear signals get through to the baby.' As we keep repeating this is one more reason to stay calm, confident and in control throughout your labour. But if you can't manage on your own this is the time when analgesics may help.

During this first stage the cervix shortens, thins and opens until it is 10 centimetres wide. There is now no division between the cervix and womb and no barrier to the baby's exit. The first stage of labour is over.

Many mothers feel ill and vomit about this time or early in the second stage. The usual causes are dehydration from over-breathing during contractions and not swallowing enough sips of water; or extreme tiredness from having a low blood sugar level. (You may be given an intravenous glucose drip to relieve this.)

Second Stage

So there you are with the baby's head pushed down through the cervix into the upper vagina. And you get an incredibly strong urge to push like hell. It's the same feeling you get when you've taken a laxative. When it works you can't fight it! In labour in exactly the same way your body tells you to push. But sometimes the midwife may not want you to. If your cervix is still not fully dilated the baby's head may be banging against a small lump of remaining cervix. If you keep pushing this lump will become tender, swollen and prolong this stage unnecessarily.

So you must wait and resist the urge to push. You can do this because in relaxation classes you learn how to pant, which cuts off the pushing instinct. When you pant your breathing sounds as if you've just finished running a 3-minute mile. The midwife will tell you when your cervix is completely opened and then you can start pushing in earnest.

Good pushing should be well controlled. It's not helpful to close your eyes, clench your fists and grunt and groan away. Again, relaxation classes teach you the correct way to push. Like this – take a very deep breath, hold it for 10 slow counts and push from the waist downwards. Then release your breath with a whoosh. See how long you can push counting backwards from 10 to 0. Long slow steady pushing is much better for the baby than short stabs at it.

You should start to push when you feel another contraction

coming on. Then you and your womb are working together to push the baby out.

The midwife will tell you just when to push – and even more important, when to stop. (You'll have been taught in relaxation classes to pant at this point since this slows down the pushing instinct.)

Walk the length of any delivery ward and you'll hear these unforgettable sounds: 'Go on, push . . . PUSH. That's it. Great, you're doing fine. Come on now, another one . . . keep going . . . go on, you can do it . . . harder . . . don't stop. And another . . . and another . . . you're nearly there . . . come on, we want to see your baby . . . PUSSSSHHHH . . .'

You may be confused at this stage because all the sensations seem to be in your back passage, not your vagina. This is because the baby is passing over your rectum. And many girls describe this phase of labour as just like being consti-pated and trying to pass a giant watermelon. That's just what having a baby really feels like. Then suddenly you feel a bulge in the vagina which is your baby's head.

As soon as you feel this wait for the next contraction and push this bulge forward. When you do this you won't feel any pain. And the delivery team will be cheering you on because they can see the baby's head appearing and disap-pearing with every push. It's a thrilling moment for your man, too, because he can see the baby's head before you can.

Episiotomy: A Short Cut?

The entrance to the vagina seems taut and over-stretched as the baby's head forces it wide open. If the skin isn't elastic enough to allow the baby through easily the doctor may decide to make a neat nick in the opening to the birth canal This is called an episiotomy – a long word for a short cut. You can't feel this because you're given a local anaesthetic. This cut is now standard practice in most hospitals and nine out of ten mums have one. It's done to prevent the skin tearing which is more difficult to stitch up and to heal than a clean, straight cut. Dissolving stitches are used in some hospitals to sew it up so there is no need to remove them later. Others use black silk which needs taking out about 6 days after the birth. (Don't worry, it's quite painless.)

After an episiotomy opens up the vaginal entrance further only one more push is needed for the baby's head to slide out. Babies normally arrive face downwards with the crown of the head uppermost. Once the head is clear it rotates so that the baby faces one of your thighs. One shoulder appears, then the other and with one final shove the baby slips out into the world with a sudden whoosh.

At last you can see your baby and find out what you've been longing to know for 9 months – whether you have a son or a daughter. And you'll hear that thrilling sound – your child's first yell proving that he or she has come bawling, battling and beautiful into our world.

In the excitement that follows you may miss the doctor cutting the baby's umbilical cord as she switches over to her own life support system and becomes an independent individual.

No matter how many times anyone witnesses this wonderful process it never fails to thrill. The parents' reaction is a happy mixture of elation, pride, tears, joy and relief, even though their newborn's wet, creased face, streaked with gunge, would be beautiful to no one else but them. Sharing this experience with your man welds loving couples together as nothing else can. For the first time a couple becomes a family.

Third Stage

You will probably be so busy admiring your baby's fantastic good looks that you won't even notice the third and last stage of labour. This is when the body painlessly expels the placenta since it is no longer needed to nourish the baby. It has done its job. Your pregnancy is over. And you're now starting the most demanding and rewarding job of your life – motherhood.

CHAPTER THIRTEEN

The Newborn

The First Hour – A Ritual of Love

Nine months of waiting, planning and dreaming result in the tiny helpless being you hold in your arms. Many hospitals hand the baby to the mother as soon as they have cleaned her face and cleared her nose and throat. But some mothers are only *shown* their babies for a few seconds before they're whisked away to a nursery. All they've seen is a little face in a tightly swaddled bundle.

The first moments of contact between baby and parents (particularly the mother) are crucial in developing a lasting emotional bond between them, psychologists now believe. American paediatrician Marshall Klaus of Case Reserve University, Cleveland, has done extensive research on this aspect of the newborn. He feels strongly that unless mothers are allowed close physical contact with their babies immediately after birth they may have trouble learning to love their children. In extreme cases this may even lead to neglect or baby battering. So the way parents meet their baby can affect them all for the rest of their lives.

Yet the love of a mother for her child – the most important in all human relationships – is the only one which begins in a strange, public place under medical supervision.

Dr. Frederick Le Boyer, a French obstetrician who in 40 years has supervised the delivery of over 10,000 babies since 1953 says: 'The first hour after birth should be set aside for a ritual of love involving mother and child.'[1] The first hour is particularly important because many babies are more responsive in the first hour after birth than at any other time in the first 24 hours of life. But we think the father should be included in this loving closeness as well. He should ask to hold his baby. And both parents should unwrap the baby together so they can cuddle and kiss her skin.

The power of a parent's loving touch works magic on a newborn baby. Research now shows that skin stimulation triggers the life force in that little body, making it more alive. So don't let anyone hurry these precious moments when you and your baby are meeting for the first time. Babies are born with an urge to respond to touch. Stroke a new baby's cheek and see how she turns her head making small sucking movements to search for a nipple.

If a mother has the chance to suckle her baby straight after birth it helps to create a stronger bond between them. It's even better if the baby suckled even before the umbilical cord is cut. Dr. Hugh Jolly says: 'God's very clever. He made umbilical cords just the right length so it's possible for babies to be lifted to the mother's breast while still connected to her body.' But of course each birth is individual and your midwife will be able to decide if this is safe for you. In most cases it will be.

But apart from the loving feeling this has physical benefits too. The suckling of the baby releases the hormone oxytocin in the mother's body. This makes the womb contract, helps to expel the placenta effortlessly and controls the bleeding. You can get the same effect by injecting a drug. But surely it's better to do this job Nature's way?

This love-in after birth is one more example of the way in which you must and can control what happens to you and your baby. Sometimes even the kindest medical staff forget the human side of childbirth because they are so involved in the technological aspect. One obstetrician told us: 'Gradually, *some* hospitals are learning that the labouring woman has feelings – and a brain she could use to help her labour and so help the hospital staff.' But this new (and welcome) attitude is still experienced by only a lucky few new mums. In most hospitals, a patient's emotional needs can be pushed into the background by hospital routine.

So stick up for your rights – but don't be bloody-minded. Hold out for the things that matter most to you. And if you feel shy or tired, remember, you're not making this effort just for your own benefit. It's vital that your baby should have a loving introduction to the world.

Special Care or Mother's Care?

One in every five babies born in Britain today goes into a Special Care unit. Often unnecessarily, says Dr. Martin Richard of the Medical Psychology Research Unit at Cambridge University. He says many babies are whisked away to these units just for observation, and not because they are suffering any serious birth complications. But who would 'observe' a new baby better than its own, eagle-eyed mother, he asks. The trouble is most of these special care units are not attached to the hospitals where the babies were born. So mother and baby are frequently separated not by glass walls but by fifty miles or more in some counties.

In a survey of 200 babies at the Royal Devon and Exeter hospital Dr. Richard found that 38 per cent did not see their mothers, apart from a brief glimpse, in their first 48 hours of life. 19 per cent had not seen either parent by the end of their first week. This separation of a baby from her parents may jeopardise their chances of forming a loving family bond, he feels.

If your baby is sent to a special care unit because she is premature or has some other serious problem you can still build a bond of love right from the start – even though this will take more planning and effort.

When you meet your baby she will probably have feeding tubes taped to her nose which won't improve her looks. Although you may not be able to hold her in your arms you can visit your baby as often as possible. Talk to her. Touch the tiny hands or stroke her skin through the windows of the incubator. Even better, ask the nurse on duty if you can do some small task for the baby – like changing a nappy.

Such small efforts may seem a poor substitute for holding

your baby and cuddling her close as you long to do, but Dr.
Richard says they have a remarkable effect. They make you
actually feel like a mother.[2] And every small task makes you
feel less helpless knowing that you are actively helping your
baby to get stronger. A premature baby usually takes around
2 years to catch up with kids who had the full 9 months in
the womb. So bear this in mind when you compare your
baby with others.

The Health Check:

In the first few days after birth the baby will be thoroughly
examined by a doctor. Her heart, breathing, colour, palate
(to make certain it's not cleft), tongue, hip joints, feet and
reflexes are all checked for normal development. The sex
organs are also carefully studied. Most new mums are surprised to find that newborns have super-sized genitals, and
often swollen breasts – in both sexes. Fathers sometimes say:
'My boy's well-endowed just like his dad!' But these en-
enlargements are caused by a hormone (produced by the
mother to stimulate the milk supply) passing through the
placenta to the baby just before birth. After a while
the swelling will subside.

A few other minor matters may worry a new mum. They
include a small swelling around the navel called a hernia, a
lopsided skull, spots, rashes, birth marks and stork bites
(turn to Chapter 26 for a fuller description of these). Then
there is the snuffling, grunting and other noisy breathing of
babies. All of these are temporary and usually disappear
without any treatment.

Jaundice:

If your baby has the St. Tropez look – the golden glow that
comes with a fortnight in the South of France – about two
days after birth, she is suffering from jaundice.

Judy:　'The last few days before my baby was born I
　　　　stuffed myself with spinach because I'd read

somewhere that it contained a special vitamin which kept a baby's blood supply free from jaundice. But two days after her arrival my daughter had a golden tan. The hospital blamed her jaundice on an incompatibility between my blood supply and hers. So I'm still wondering about the magic of spinach.'

Jaundice is usually quite harmless and vanishes after a few days. Severe cases are treated by putting the baby's crib under a special light with her eyes covered to protect them from the glare. If this happens to your baby visit her as often as possible and hold her hands while you talk to her so that your baby feels your presence and is comforted. When jaundice is present at birth it's more serious and the baby may need a blood transfusion.

Many doctors now believe there is a link between induced births and jaundice in the newborn. A study in the North of England by Dr. John Beazley and Dr. Brian Alderman found that the more Oxytocin hormone used to induce or speed up labour the more likely a baby would suffer from jaundice. Other doctors simply blame the jaundice on the high number of red cells which break down rapidly in the blood supply after birth. And the yellow pigment called bilirubin in these cells gives the skin its golden tinge.[3]

Some hospitals believe that lots of liquid, like boiled cooled water helps to clean the baby's blood supply and so cure the jaundice. But the Royal Worcester Infirmary has had wonderful results by allowing jaundiced babies to breast feed on demand as long as they like. In this case mother's milk seems more effective.

Squinting:

All newborn babies squint at some time or other. This is because their eye muscles are still weak. Any squint should be cured by six months. If it's not tell your doctor because early treatment is essential.

Circumcision:

Some parents think it is cleaner and healthier for a baby boy to be circumcised. This means the removal of the foreskin covering the tip of the penis. But this surgery is not necessary and not usually performed nowadays except for religious reasons. Both the Jewish and Moslem faiths require this.

The Navel:

The stump of the umbilical cord always gives new mums a bit of worry when caring for their babies. Hospitals tell you simply to keep it clean and sprinkle it with antiseptic powder which they supply. It usually dries up and falls off within a week or two. Sometimes a few spots of blood appear when this happens but they're nothing to worry about.

Guthrie Test:

Before the baby leaves the hospital he will be given the Guthrie test. This is a standard procedure. A minute blood sample is taken from her heel to test for any inherited diseases which could slow the baby's mental development. Such defects are rare but may be cured with a special diet if discovered in time. That's why this test is so important.

Registration:

Most large maternity hospitals have a visiting registrar who tours the wards so that new parents can register the birth of their babies. If the baby is born at home you or your man must visit the nearest registry office (your local Town Hall will give you its address) within 42 days of the birth (21 in Scotland).

You can get two versions of a birth certificate – plain and fancy. The simple one simply states the baby's name, date and place of birth. It may be more suitable for an unmarried mother. And even for married mums it has another advantage – it doesn't state your age! The fuller certificate listing all relevant details can be bought if you wish.

The First Week

You'll spend a lot of the first week just looking at your baby,
double-checking that she really is in beautiful condition.
New mum nerves are understandable especially if this is
your first child. Remember, one result of today's smaller
family units is only about 10 per cent of women have had any
experience of handling small babies before they have their
own.

This is why you may not instantly feel like a born mother.
Don't worry about it. Dr. Hugh Jolly told a gathering of
mums from all over Britain: 'I'd like to see a notice in every
maternity ward saying, "You may have fallen in love with
your husband at first sight. Or it might have taken time to fall
in love with him. It may also take time to fall in love with
your baby". The myth of instant motherhood must go. Most
mums have muddled feelings and these should be recognised
by the hospital staff.' (*See* page 178.)

First Feeding:

Sometimes to give you a good rest hospital staff will suggest
they give the baby a bottle for her first feed after birth. But
if you want to breast feed the sooner you start the better.
Most babies have a strong impulse to suck at birth, and if
they don't get the chance fairly soon, they may lose interest.
So when you go to sleep remind the nurse on duty that you
want to be woken to feed your baby yourself. (For more on
breastfeeding *see* Chapter 15.)

Milk Rash:

A few weeks after birth your baby's face may become dotted
with white spots. Usually these appear just when lots of
visitors are eager to see the new arrival and you want her to
look her best. But you should not try to squeeze or otherwise
deal with these spots. They are called milk spots because it
was once believed that they were a sign that the baby's milk

disagreed with her. Their medical name is milia and they are caused by blocked oil glands in the skin. Without any treatment they will disappear.

'Stork Bites':

These are the red patches which appear on newborn babies most commonly on or around the eyes and the back of the neck. Don't worry about them as they fade after a few months.

The Fontanelles:

At birth your baby's head has not finished growing. This is the reason you'll find a soft section on top of her scalp which has no bone beneath. It's called a fontanelle and you may see the heartbeat pulsing under the skin. But don't worry, it's perfectly normal. After about 18 months the forebones of the skull will be knitted together. Parents often worry about hurting the baby through the fontanelle but there is a really tough membrane as thick as workmen's denim jeans protecting the gap. You may find another soft spot at the back of her skull but this is usually knitted together by birth or soon afterwards.

Weight Loss:

Don't worry if your baby loses weight in the first few days of life. All newborns lose about 10 per cent of their birth weight. The larger the baby the more she is likely to lose. The bottle fed baby will take 2 or 3 days before her digestive system is working well. And a breastfed baby even longer, because her mother's milk does not start flowing for several days after the birth. Until the milk arrives the baby sucks colostrum, a thicker yellow liquid which is extremely nourishing and gives the baby protection from many diseases the mother has had.

The Other End:

Even if your baby hasn't been fed since birth she will need a nappy change in the first 6–12 hours of life. Her first stools will be meconium, a greenish-black gunge. But you won't have to hold your nose because it doesn't smell. Hospital staff will note the time this happens. But after a few days the colour changes to yellow and remains soft, especially if she is breast fed.

Twin Births:

Two babies at once doubles the work but also the delights of being parents. However multiple births are becoming rarer – despite the growing use of fertility drugs. Only 1 in a 100 births produces more than one baby today, whereas in the 1950s the rate was 1.3 in 100.

Research shows that the chances of a multiple birth rise the more children a woman has and the older she is. But as women have babies younger today and have smaller families, twins and triplets are now less common.

Twins may be fraternal or identical. The first kind are the result of fertilisation of two separate eggs by separate sperm about the same time. And so they have separate placentas in the womb. And the babies resemble each other no more than any other children of the same family.

Identical twins are produced by one egg dividing into two and they share a single placenta in the womb.

A mother expecting twins needs more rest than usual to cope with the extra demands on her body. And her babies may be premature simply because two babies soon outgrow the space for one in the womb.

It's quite possible to breast feed twins as the supply of breast milk always equals the demand. One baby is often more placid than the other and may wait her turn. Or a dummy will comfort a more demanding twin. But you can breast feed both at the same time. A health visitor's advice and help are invaluable to the mother of twins. She can also suggest ways to plan your schedule to give both babies equal love and attention.

Bathing:

Memories are made at bath time. The sight of a slippery, soapy little body with wet curls and the sound of delighted gurgles as little hands splash in the water is one of parents' fondest memories.

Yet bath time can be a nightmare in the early weeks, especially for a new mother. Unused to handling such a tiny creature she is terrified of dropping the baby. And unsure of the right way to do the bath procedure she was shown in the maternity hospital.

Val: 'Baths were something I dreaded in the early days. I had visions of the baby slipping from my lap, sliding on to the floor and cracking her skull. Of course, it never happened. But the thought kept me tense and unhappy. Moreover the baby screamed from the start of the bath till the end. Then an experienced friend who saw this unhappy scene gave me two of the best tips I ever had. She told me the baby was screaming because she was hungry. I had been warned never to bath after a feed. "Nonsense", said my friend. "Feed her, then wait a quarter of an hour. Then have a nice relaxed time with your baby."

'All went just as she predicted. The other tip came when she saw how diffident I was about soaping the baby on my shaky lap. She said: "Don't bother. The baby isn't dirty. She just needs to be refreshed. Simply dunk her into soapy water, play with her and make sure you carefully wipe the nappy area dry." Those two tips took the agony out of baths for my baby and me. When I became more used to handling her I did the correct bathing routine just as the hospital taught me. But I did it when I was ready.'

CHAPTER FOURTEEN

Days of Milk and Roses

If you want to know how it feels to be a superstar, have a baby. Sitting up in bed surrounded by flowers, well-wishers, telegrams and cards is a blissful feeling. The compliments showered on you and your baby's beauty keep you on this bubbly high for days. You don't get quite the same excitement with a second baby so make the most of it. And remember, a maternity ward is one place where hospital staff shut their eyes to the alcohol consumed on the premises!

Val: 'I was lucky enough to be sent a bottle of champagne by the editor of the newspaper I then worked on. The card sent with it read: "For post-natal dyspepsia. One glassful every half hour." Needless to say, the medicine was taken.'

The Hospital Co-op

The secret of true happiness in hospital is to make friends with the other mothers and – just as important – with the nurses. It won't be difficult because you all have something wonderful in common. For up to 10 days you'll have fun being totally single-minded about your favourite subjects – the birth and the beauty of your baby.

But this fun time is no rest cure. Annie, a girl we know, saw the sourest sister in her ward smile once. That was when she noticed a bundle of books and magazines Annie had taken to hospital, 'When do you think you'll get time to read those?' she laughed. And the waspish nurse was right.

Annie was much too busy to lie in bed reading all day. You'll be surprised how much you have to fit into one ordinary hospital day.

Between your meals, the baby's feeds, nappy changes, doctor's visits, your baths and freshening-up sessions, you end up with precious little time to relax. Any spare moments left outside visiting hours, are taken up with writing thank-you letters or sneaking in extra salt baths to ease the discomfort of those stitches. (You'll find it difficult to walk for the first few days after the birth because of them.)

Your day may begin soon after 5 a.m. and end around 10 p.m. And after the first few nights, you'll be expected to wake for your baby's 2 a.m. feed. So your hospital stay is far from a lovely, lazy rest. Incidentally, you could also be troubled with 'after-pains': when the womb is contracting after the baby's birth there may be some discomfort. Some women have more after-pains than others. Usually, a pain killer is all you need for these.

New Mum Nerves

Handling your baby for the first few days can also be re-assuring when you know that every new mum is feeling the way you do: petrified. But there's a great spirit we call the hospital co-op in some wards where all the new mums rally around to give each other confidence and help.

Judy: 'I watched a mum in the bed opposite me, change her baby from top to tail. Just as she was fastening his nappy, he squirted her straight in the eye and wet himself all over again. His mother sat down and wailed: "I give up. I think I'll send him back." And she wasn't joking. Her eyes were brimming as she sat down again, too tired to cope. But the rest of us went to her aid. One girl lent her a clean nappy and vest, another changed the crib's under-sheet and a third asked for first refusal if the baby was really for sale. Two days later, when she was feeling stronger, this "hopeless" mum was the first to help another mum in trouble.'

After the birth and the baby, your third biggest talking point in the hospital ward is your bowels! It's not easy after stitches and labour to do any hard pressing in the lavatory. Not surprisingly, bowel movements (or rather, the lack of them) become incredibly important with anxious daily queries from nurses. One of us was in a ward with a Canadian mum who was sitting hopefully in the lavatory one day – with the tap running so that the sound of water would encourage her – when she was interrupted. Her mother was on the phone, from Toronto. 'Just like Mother,' she commented afterwards. 'She *always* interrupts at the most inconvenient moments!'

Wouldn't it be a good idea for N.H.S. hospitals to serve wholewheat bread and Muesli for breakfast instead of the corn flakes and white plastic bread they give you now? Apart from being healthier food, these would save the expense of suppositories and other laxatives. So the added expense of the natural foods might be covered. (If you are constipated, ask friends to bring you lots of fresh fruit which may do the trick more naturally than medicine.)

After Birth

After the delivery, some new mums' pregnancy problems are not quite over. One or more of several hassles could make you feel a bit fragile. Every new mum has a vaginal flow called the lochia. This is just like the flow of a normal period but may last longer – anywhere from one to five weeks. Avoid the risk of infection, doctors suggest, by using external sanitary towels instead of tampons and these may be kinder to your episiotomy stitches as well. If you have a tender seat, as a result of the stitches or pregnancy piles, ask the nurse for a rubber ring to make sitting in bed more comfortable. A few mums may find that when their milk starts – a few days after birth – that their breasts become engorged, turning rock-hard and sometimes very painful. The nurses will help you – the solution is usually to squeeze a little milk out of the breasts before starting to feed. This relieves the built-up pressure but applying hot towels will help and so will the hospital's breast pump.

Pulling Together

In some ways hospital routine reminds you of schooldays with lights out at 10 and other rules and regulations. But doing boring work together makes it more fun. For example, at some time during your hospital stay a bossy lady physio-therapist (they're always bossy) comes round to teach you post-natal exercises. These help to pull your innards back together and banish the pregnant lady's swayback.

Doing these exercises is important because they not only help your figure but your sex life too. Unfortunately so many new mums don't bother doing the exercises then moan later that having a child has made their bladders dribble if they so much as cough or sneeze. (If this is your problem drink four glasses of water to flush out the bladder.) So doing these exercises regularly is vitally important. In the ward goody-goodies can egg slackers on, remind each other how the exercises are done – and then do them at one special time each day, say mid-morning.

We found that if you call them sexercises and emphasise how much they improve your love life more girls are keen to do them (and keep doing them at home afterwards).

Father's Hour

Your most important visitor is the baby's father. Hospitals which set aside one visiting hour each day for fathers only know what they're doing. You do need to be protected from too many well-wishers because they can exhaust you. More important, visitors take the emphasis away from the father. He can rightly feel neglected and vulnerable because everyone he knows seems to be concentrating on the mother and the baby. And no one likes being pushed into the background.

There are ways that a BabyLove mum can minimise this feeling. When father arrives for visiting hours don't greet him sitting up in bed with your baby in your arms like a Lady Madonna. Leave the baby in her crib so that your arms are free to hug him. Being alone together to chat quietly makes a soothing oasis in the usual hubbub of hospital activity. And your baby's father will feel your love for him hasn't changed, even though he has to share it from now on with someone else.

A divorcee we know says her marriage first went wrong at the maternity home where she had her daughter. She told us: 'I can see clearly now that it's too late that from the beginning I concentrated too much on the baby. When my husband visited me in hospital I always had the baby in my arms. I talked about little else and obviously showed that I cared about nothing else.'

Birth of the Blues

A few days after your baby's birth you may suddenly notice a lot of red-eyed ladies in your ward making tissue manufacturers rich. Tears are a natural come-down after the highly emotional experience of giving birth. They're caused by the sudden hormonal changes in your body as it returns to its pre-pregnancy state. The weepy feeling doesn't last very long, it happens to most women, and the best way to get through it is to have a good, long cry. Bottling it up only prolongs the agony. You may understand the reasons for it more easily if you remember this: periods often make women moody and upset. So giving birth is much more likely to make you unstable and teary. It's nice to know

CHAPTER FIFTEEN

Everything You Didn't Think You'd Need To Know About Feeding Your Baby

When feeding your baby you're not just supplying her with nourishment, you're also filling her up with love. So it seems amazing that mothers used to feed their babies by the clock and not when the baby's hunger cries told them.

We've heard stories from older relatives, of women who used to stand outside the baby's room listening to the frantic screams within. They'd dig their nails into their palms waiting until the clock ticked on to the hour specified for feeding by some expert. Meanwhile, their breasts would be aching while milk dripped down to stain the fronts of their blouses.

Horrific tales like this are unknown today, thank goodness. (At least, they should be.) Modern mums know that feeding to a strict time-table is unkind to babies whose appetites vary just as adults' do. Almost every baby quickly settles into a reasonable routine, feeding roughly every four hours. But this schedule will be her own, not arranged by some baby expert on the other side of the world.

Remember, babies don't understand that the rest of us live by clocks and routines. A baby who's hungry is really ravenous and if left to wait, may develop stomach pains. The younger she is, the less she's able to wait. By crying for food she uses up energy she needs to suckle. The result is when she is finally fed she is too tired to feed properly. Then her mother thinks: 'What's all the fuss about? She wasn't really hungry at all.' And she tells everyone she has a difficult baby.

Like everything else in caring for your child, a baby's

needs *must* come first. So if she cries for her dinner, drop what you're doing and feed her at once. Let her tummy tell you the right feeding time. One day it may be 11.30 a.m., the next 12.15 p.m. This is called demand feeding.

But Dr. Hugh Jolly begs people not to use the phrase 'demand feeding'. He prefers to call it 'ask' feeding because he says too many mothers are afraid they can't cope with a baby's demands.[1] But whatever you call it, a BabyLove mum knows there's no other way.

Breast Feeding:

Breast feeding is the most loving way a mother can feed her baby. Snuggling into the bosom restores the closeness that the baby lost on leaving the womb. Remember, for the first nine months of life your baby has been a part of you. Now you've been suddenly separated, but through breast feeding this closeness is restored regularly throughout the day and night. These special times together may some day be consciously forgotten but the emotional link they create can never be erased.

Bottle fed babies may also be cuddled during feeding but layers of clothes separate them from this vital contact with their mother's skin. Nevertheless, bottle feeding is the popular way to feed a baby in most of the Western World today. In Britain only one-third of mothers even make an attempt to breast feed. One month later only half this number still have a baby at the breast. And only a tiny proportion of babies are still being breast fed at the age of 3 months.

To us this seems not just sad but worrying. Overwhelming evidence – including the latest Government report on child nutrition – confirms that breast is best – for a mother as well as her baby.

Quite apart from the benefits to your baby's emotional health, the chief argument in favour of breast feeding is safety. Breast fed babies rarely become cot death victims.

Research into unexplained infant deaths points to bottled baby milk being a major cause. Doctors think one reason could be tiny sensing devices in a baby's throat. These check the milk that flows over them. When a baby is fed its mother's milk there is no reaction. But when cow's milk is swallowed these sensing devices can depress the baby's breathing.

With bottle feeds there is a danger of mixing too-strong a milk formula (the 'one for the pot' syndrome), even when made up to the manufacturer's precise instructions. Over-strong milk mixtures can lead to dehydration of a baby's body, also linked with cot deaths. Cow's milk has a higher salt level than breast milk and this puts an extra load on a baby's kidneys. Fewer breast fed babies get stomach infections such as gastro-enteritis. And they are less likely to get fat because breast milk has fewer calories.

But apart from the loving closeness and safety, breast feeding has a lot more advantages. It's the first and greatest of all convenience foods. In the middle of a cold winter night there's no need to stagger downstairs to a chilly kitchen to get a bottle of milk and then serve it at the right temperature.

Breast milk is ready on tap in the most beautiful package, with a teat which just naturally fits into a baby's mouth. The milk flows the way your baby needs it – fast at first when the baby is hungriest, then slower. And all this doesn't cost you a penny. Best of all, while the mother's milk is good nourishment for your baby breast feeding helps your body too. The suckling action of the baby makes the womb contract and helps it to shrink back to normal size much faster.

Your body expects you to breast feed. The milk supply must be forced to dry up if you don't. Even if you breast feed for just a week you'll be giving your baby a better start in life. During the first days after birth your breasts produce a thick, creamy yellow substance called colostrum. This is very high in protein and passes on to your baby the immunity you have to certain diseases. There's no artificial equivalent of colostrum so if you skip breast feeding your baby misses out on this vital protection in the all-important first days of life.

6 Questions every Woman Wants to ask about Breast Feeding

1 Q: *Does it hurt?*
  A: To be truthful, yes, in the first days after you begin to breast feed you will feel a sharp nip as the baby's gums clamp down around the nipple. This only lasts a second or two and is quickly followed by a soothing sensation. After a week or two you won't even feel this little pang. Special nipple creams which you can buy at chemists do help if applied after feeds.

2 Q: *Do you need big breasts?*
  A: Neither your nipples nor your breasts need be big. In fact, small breasted women often have more milk because their breasts have less fatty tissue.

3 Q: *How will I know if the baby is getting enough?*
  A: You can't tell how much milk the baby has swallowed. But if she drops off to sleep contentedly after being fed and wakes up about the right time for her next feed you don't have a thing to worry about. A baby gets all the nourishment she needs within the first 3 minutes of sucking. After that she suckles for comfort and pleasure.

4 Q: *Will I feel like a cow?*
  A: Some women think they will until they actually begin breast feeding. Doing what comes naturally makes you far less like a milking machine and much more like a real woman. Many women discover great physical pleasure in breast feeding and hate weaning their babies.

5 Q: *Do you need a special diet while breast feeding?*
  A: No, but a well-balanced diet, low on starches and high on protein, vitamins and minerals is as good for breast feeding as it is for regaining your figure. It may be a good idea to avoid highly spiced foods like curry

which could disagree with the baby. But a little of what you fancy won't do any harm.

6 Q: *Will it make me flat-chested?*
   A: It's pregnancy not breast feeding which is mainly responsible for any change in your bust measurement. So you won't have a better outline by bottle feeding.

Breast Feeding and Sex

Breast feeding makes you more sexy, believe it or not! Doctors say it brings back that loving feeling to a woman far quicker than if she bottle fed. A study of American mothers showed that those who breast fed wanted to make love after childbirth much sooner than those who didn't. So as well as benefiting you and your baby, breast feeding is also indirectly great for your man! And maybe directly, too. American anthropologist Ashley Montagu, author of *Touching* says: 'Men who have not been breast fed make lousy lovers. If one doesn't learn about touching and response at the mother's breast, then the prospect of ever learning is abysmal – particularly for males because females can compensate later on. Little girls always get a great deal more touching from their parents when they're growing up so they can more readily recoup the loss. Little boys can't. Therefore, unless a man has been breast fed he will always be handicapped as a result.'[2]

A lot of men enjoy watching their wives breast feed because just by being there, they share in the fulfilment this gives a woman. As one man who wished his wife could go on breast feeding forever told us: 'It was a living picture of everything womanly.'

Although most women don't think of breast feeding in a sexual way a few do admit feeling sexually excited by it. (A small minority claim they were so aroused that they reached a climax.) Women with this sensual experience may be shocked and think it unnatural so they guiltily give up and switch to bottle feeding. The reason for this may be connected with the belief that breasts are only meant for sexual purposes – the result of brainwashing by mass media and the advertising world. This may also be one reason why some men object to their wives breast feeding.

Unfortunately, this conditioning goes so deep that many women may shrink from an experience which could give them so much deep enjoyment. The situation is not improved by the public taboo on breast feeding in public. People who think like this should remember that breasts were used for feeding long before they were used to advertise motor cars.

The Anti-Breast Feeders

Some people find breast feeding a beautiful experience, others think it turns them into human cows. But can you know your feelings in advance? We say: 'Don't knock it until you've tried it.' Your attitude may completely change once you do. But if you're one of those ladies who can't even bear the thought, don't force yourself.

Your unwillingness can be sensed by your baby because even the tiniest newborn is highly sensitive to her mother's feelings. (When you're depressed and low your baby will reflect your mood and 'act up'. Then see how she changes when you feel better.)

Val: 'In Israel, hospitals are so keen on breast feeding they don't allow patients any choice. All mums are required to breast feed. One result of this policy was a mother I met on a trip out there who confessed to me that because she loathed breast feeding she had grown to dislike her baby son. This feeling changed when she switched to bottle feeding once she'd left hospital. But even now, 2 years later, when her son cries in the night and she goes to him, he cries louder for his dad. She thinks the only reason is the bad start they had together.'

Breast feeding only works if the mother's attitude is right. If it's not, the body produces an adverse reaction which cuts down your milk supply, so the baby doesn't get enough milk and needs a supplement of bottled milk. And the more you bottle feed the less milk your breasts produce.

Don't persevere with breast feeding unless you really want to. A tense unhappy mother will result in a tense, unhappy baby. And feeding times will turn into a battle – within yourself, as well as with the baby – instead of a relaxed time which you'll both enjoy.

How to Breast Feed

The size of your breasts is not as important as the shape of your nipples. If they don't stick out nicely from the surrounding dark area called the areola, the baby may find sucking difficult. So examine your nipples to see if they can do the job. But don't be too worried if they are flat or inverted. You can buy nipple shields to draw them out and if you have any doubts, always ask your doctor.

Around the time you're about 4 or 5 months pregnant it helps if you give your breasts a little squeeze now and then to get a drop of fluid from the nipples. Or tweak them when you are lying in the bath. The warmth of the water and this stimulation helps to clear the milk ducts. But this preparation isn't essential. And if you have a sensitive, sexy husband, he'll do the job for you!

Before putting the baby to the breast you should wash your nipple to ward off any infection. Then make certain that the baby takes all the dark areola, not just the nipple, into her mouth. Your milk flows fastest when the baby is hungriest, in the first three minutes of feeding. The remainder of the time your baby is not only gaining comfort but the suckling motion which is stronger at your breast than on a bottle, helps develop the baby's jaws, palate and throat muscles. This sucking action also pulls your womb back into normal shape, too. You can feel it contract while you feed.

Many experts still say you should time your baby's feeds, building up to a maximum of 10 minutes and no more. But several enlightened doctors now think that mums should forget about clockwatching when feeding. A baby should feed as long as it likes – within reason. If you find your baby wants to spend 24 hours a day glued to your nipples maybe you should buy a dummy. Obviously she enjoys being comforted this way (*see* page 199 for more information on pacifiers).

You'll find it easier to open a sleepy baby's mouth by pressing your index finger firmly on her chin. Her mouth will drop open automatically. And if her face is turned away from your nipple, simply tickle the nearest cheek with your finger. Her mouth will immediately turn towards you.

Judy: 'I was taught to breast feed a baby for exactly 3 minutes for the first few days. When this time was up the nurse showed me how to slip my little finger into the corner of the baby's mouth and pull her off the nipple. I found out too late that this was the worst thing I could have done. Within 48 hours I had such a badly cracked nipple that I had to use a nipple shield and a breast pump. Dragging the baby's mouth off the breast in this way caused the crack. And each feed made it worse. Within 2 weeks I had the beginning of a painful breast abscess.'

Like anything new, practice makes it easier and you'll soon get the knack of it. You can protect your nipples from cracks and infection by massaging them with a special breast cream available from chemists. You should always discuss any problems with your health visitor.

What if you're worried that the baby isn't getting enough food? This is one of the main problems mums encounter when breast feeding. We think one top London paediatrician has the right answer. He says: 'Doctors are always joking that they'll have to invent a transparent breast so mothers can see exactly how much milk has flowed into the baby. I'd rather invent opaque feeding bottles. The greatest mistake every mother makes in bottle feeding is hoping her baby will finish the bottle. But the baby may finish it just to please his mother, and become fat by swallowing more than he needs.'

Babies aren't naturally greedy. So don't worry that your baby doesn't seem to be taking much milk. As long as she's gaining weight steadily – around 6 ounces a week – and seems content, she's doing fine.

It would be a little pious to suggest that you should never sneak a peek at television or read a book while breast feeding. But when you look down at your feeding baby you'll notice that her eyes rarely leave your face. So why not give her that same loving attention?

How to Wean

Only you can decide when to stop breast feeding. It depends on whether you have to be a working mum and how soon your baby gets teeth. A sharp nip from a new incisor may make up your mind, though many mums say that teething doesn't really interfere with breast feeding. And lots of women enjoy breast feeding so much they go on as long as possible. A social worker we know recalls a time when she called at a house and saw a mother still breast feeding her 4-year-old daughter. 'Isn't it time you weaned her?' she suggested. Before the mother could reply, the little girl piped up: 'Mind your own business!'

You should start weaning gradually. Begin by dropping one feed – probably a daytime one around 2 p.m. or 6 p.m. and substitute this with bottled baby milk. 2 or 3 days later leave out a morning one as well and offer a bottle instead (or a cup if your baby is old enough). You may have trouble persuading a baby to take milk from a bottle because she's so used to the warmth and comfort of your breast.

Val: 'The first time I offered my baby a bottle of milk she screamed and wouldn't even try it. After half an hour in desperation I phoned my local branch of the National Childbirth Trust who have a special breast feeding advisory service. The lady on duty told me my daughter was being very intelligent. "She can smell your milk and can't understand why you're fobbing her off with something else." Her solution? "Put the baby and the bottle in her father's loving arms and disappear." I did this and the little guzzler swallowed every drop without a fuss.'

Breast Feeding in Public

If anyone sees you breast feeding and objects it's their attitude that's wrong, not yours. It's a pity that the sight of a naked breast in some newspapers and magazines is acceptably naughty but a breast feeding mother is obscene. We think the real obscenity is in the minds of the onlooker who turns a beautiful, natural act into something shameful.

21 Ways to Compare Feeding Methods

Breast Feeding	*Bottle Feeding*
1 Mother's milk designed for babies	Cow's milk designed for calves
2 Costs nothing	Costs rise regularly
3 Instantly available at correct temperature	Needs exact preparation and you may have to wait until it cools
4 More hygienic so less likely to cause infection	Inexact preparation linked with stomach infections like gastro-enteritis, convulsions and even cot deaths

5 Producing milk burns up calories – you regain your figure faster	Figure not affected
6 Closer contact with mother	Contact more with bottle than mum
7 Container designed by Nature to suit baby	Container mass produced and may not suit every baby
8 Less likely to make baby fat, containing fewer calories	Can cause excess weight if milk not made up exactly to manufacturer's instructions
9 Flows fastest when baby hungriest at start of feed	Flows at same rate throughout
10 Night feeds on tap	Night feeds may be a lot of bother
11 More pleasant nappy changes as stool less smelly and less chance of nappy rash	Bowel motions firmer, may be more frequent, more smelly, higher risk of nappy rash
12 No stock of food necessary for travelling	Lots of equipment needed even on shortest journey
13 Quality of product constant	Might have difficulty finding your brand. Supplies can be irregular at local shop
14 Suits baby until weaned	May need switching from one brand to another until most suitable found
15 Protein-rich colostrum in vital first days gives mother's immunities to baby	You can't buy colostrum or anything similar

16 Cannot know baby's exact intake	You know precisely amount swallowed
17 No one else can feed baby unless you take the trouble to express milk from breast into bottle	Family may enjoy feeding baby
18 Tiredness or illness can affect milk supply	Your health has no effect on milk
19 Painkillers and other drugs can pass through milk to baby	Your diet doesn't affect milk
20 Nipple problems or breast infections can interfere with feeding	Mother's body doesn't affect milk
21 Public feeding may be embarrassing to you or others	No problem with feeding in public

Bottle Feeding

If for some reason you can't breast feed, your baby needn't lose out on love or proper nourishment. As bottle feeding is the most popular way to feed babies today it's obvious that children can survive and thrive beautifully on it. Probably a lot of bonny baby contest-winners and quiz kids were raised this way. And it didn't do them any harm.

The main reservation we have about bottle feeding is that mother and baby could lose the warm skin-on-skin closeness that comes naturally with breast feeding. There is a nice way you can make up for this if you really believe *very* strongly that it's a vital early lesson in love. Here's how:

An advocate of natural motherhood, after years of helping

new mums, advises them to undo their bras while bottle feeding. In this way the mother feels closer to her baby and can make direct skin contact.[3]

However you go about it, our only feeding rule is: what you feed your baby is secondary to the way you do it.

Choosing a milk

The shelves in chemist shops are crammed with dozens of different types and brands of artificial baby milks. So choosing the right one can be very confusing. Most milks are based on cow's milk and come in 2 main forms – powdered or liquid, although this is not yet generally available. (Some mothers use evaporated or condensed milk but we don't recommend them. Condensed milk is much too sugary and evaporated is not as close to mother's milk as powdered or liquid kinds.)

Ordinary cow's milk is totally unsuitable for young babies. It has less carbohydrate (sugars and starches) than breast milk but twice as much protein and about 4 times as much of some minerals. So cow's milk must be modified to make it suitable for small babies. More carbohydrate is added and the protein and mineral content reduced.

We think the main points to consider in choosing an artificial milk are:

1 Is it the closest equivalent to mother's milk? (ask your health visitor to advise you about this).

2 Is it easy to prepare? (concentrated liquid milks are the simplest and therefore safest).

3 How much does it cost? (after you have found a suitable brand watch out for the prices merry-go-round. It may be on special offer in your chemist shop one week and reduced at the supermarket the next. But the cheapest price of all should be at your baby health clinic).

Equipment:

This is thoroughly covered in Chapter 8.

How to start:

Every good mum will be as clean as she is careful when
preparing a baby's feeds. It's no good being slap-dash about
hygiene. Giving your hands a quick rinse under a cold tap
then wiggling your fingers in the air to dry them just isn't
safe enough. You may think a few germs don't matter but
you'll think differently if your baby gets a stomach infection.

So always begin by being pernickety. Wash your hands
with hot soapy water and dry them thoroughly. Make sure
all work surfaces are not only clean but dry. Sterilise everything that comes into contact with your baby's food. This
includes the knife used to level off scoops of powder, and the
jug feeds are mixed in.

All this cleanliness is necessary because milk is a great
breeding ground for bacteria and these germs multiply
quickly at room temperature (that's why feeds must be
stored in a refrigerator).

There are two chief ways to sterilise:

1 Boiling: Everything you need should be completely
submerged in water which is then brought to the
boil, and kept bubbling for between 5 and 10
minutes.

2 Soaking: This is now an easier and more popular way to
sterilise feeding equipment. You submerge the
equipment in water, just as for boiling. Then
add a liquid sterilising solution or tablet in
amounts directed by the manufacturer. This
solution must be changed every 24 hours.

Making up feeds:

If your baby is completely bottle fed it is easier to make up a
whole day's supply of bottles in one batch. Then you can
store them in the fridge and take one out as needed. Preparing these every day is a boring grind. However there are a
few golden rules in safe preparation which you must *never*
break. Your baby's health is at risk if you do.

1 Follow the manufacturer's directions *exactly*. Adding an extra scoop of powder like one-for-the-pot is dangerous. If you have any difficulty ask your health visitor about it.

2 Always use boiling water which has been allowed to cool. Boiling water destroys the precious vitamin content and can make the feed lumpy and harder to blend.

3 Don't try to economise by adding too much water. Or by saving left-over feeds from one day to the next.

How to bottle feed:

Cradle the baby in your arms keeping her head raised. This is important because if the baby lies flat there is a danger that milk may run back up the tubes leading from the throat to the middle ear, and this may lead to ear infections. This is also the reason a baby should never be left on its own with a propped bottle.

A hungry baby will open her mouth when she feels the bottle near her mouth and begin sucking strongly. Keep the bottle tilted so that the teat is always filled with milk. This prevents the baby swallowing air at the same time as milk.

The baby will feel more comfortable if you gently pull back on the bottle. This stops the full weight of the milk-filled bottle resting on the baby's mouth and helps her to suck more easily.

If the baby cries during feeding shake some drops out of the teat on to your hand to check that the hole in the teat isn't blocked.

Other drinks:

When a baby cries many mothers automatically think she is hungry and offer her a drink of milk. But babies can get thirsty just like adults. And between feeds it is better to offer your baby boiled cooled water to which a few drops of orange juice, rose hip syrup or other fruit juice has been added.

Extra fluids are especially important if the baby is sick to avoid dehydration. Talk to your baby clinic or health visitor about this.

Vitamins:

Your health visitor or baby clinic will sell you at a very low reduced price a bottle of vitamin drops. The baby needs these in increasing amounts every day until she is 5 years old.

Babies need extra vitamins because they are growing faster at this time than any other in their lives. But giving young babies vitamin drops can be difficult. If you add the drops to a bottle you can't be certain the baby will receive the full dose. Some of the drops may cling to the sides of the bottle. So put the drops on the tip of a small plastic spoon and gently pour them into the baby's mouth. If you are breast feeding you may find it works better to put the vitamins one drop at a time on the tip of a nipple.

Is She Still Hungry?

Always prepare a little more milk than you estimate the baby wants. Then if her appetite grows, she'll drink the extra milk. And if not, she'll leave it in the bottle.

Babies always stop feeding when they've had enough. Most start with 6 feeds of 4 to 5 ounces of milk per feed. But the amount she wants depends on her weight. Doctors calculate a healthy baby needs $2\frac{1}{2}$ fluid ounces per pound per day. If you have trouble calculating the correct amount, it's important to check with your health visitor.

Dropping Night Feeds

As your baby grows larger and heavier, she will stop needing night feeds. Some babies first sleep through the 2 a.m. feed while others drop the 10 p.m. one first. But babies don't suddenly drop night feeding habits. You may find that instead of waking as usual at 2 a.m., your baby will sleep through to 3 a.m. or even 4 a.m. If that happens, feed her when she wakes and treat it as the 2 a.m. usual feed. Around four hours later, she may feel hungry again and wake. The

next night, she may sleep until 5 a.m. or revert to waking at
2 a.m. If you are demand feeding, you'll feed whenever
your baby needs it. But don't jump out of bed at the first
little wail. She just may change her mind and go back to
sleep. The 10 p.m. or evening feed can be handled the same
way. Need we add that any mother who wakes her baby for a
feed is a crazy lady who loves creating problems for herself.
Her baby may be ready to sleep through the night if only her
mum would let her!

Is Burping Necessary?

It's part of the feeding ritual: first you feed your baby and
then you burp her. But is burping really necessary? New
thinking suggests that millions of mothers have wasted
precious sleeping hours waiting for that magic burp to rise.
Doctors now say that if your baby cries while being burped
half-way through a feed, it's probably not because she has
wind. It's just that she's hungry and hates being interrupted!

Wind is hardly ever a cause of a baby's crying says top
London paediatrician, Hugh Jolly. You're wasting valuable
sleeping time if you sit for hours trying to burp your baby in
the middle of the night. (The baby doesn't mind how much
sleep you lose – she probably loves having her back rubbed.)
Of course, burping doesn't do any harm but struggling to
bring up wind only makes mothers and babies exhausted.
Despite this, if you feel you absolutely *must* burp, this is the
easy BabyLove way to do it. Sit the baby on your lap. Rest
her chin on the thumb and forefinger of your right hand.
Then raise her chin so that the windpipe in the throat forms a
straight line to the chest. Now the air passages are clear and
the wind can rise – if there's any down there.

CHAPTER SIXTEEN

Early Days and Late Nights

As a new mum you should really get a week alone in a luxury hotel, complete with 'Do not disturb' sign on your bedroom door. You actually *need* this rest – but you can't have it because caring for your baby means you're on call 24 hours a day, 7 days a week, 52 weeks of the year with no time off for good behaviour. (These anti-social hours prompted one new mum we know to joke weakly to her husband after a particularly tiring day with her 3-week-old son: 'Do you think it's *really* too late for an abortion?')

The joy of arriving home with your baby is mixed with a few little shocks to the system. During the first few days, you'll suddenly reach for a clean nappy – and find your supply is almost gone. In the corner, is a rapidly growing pile of soiled baby linen which won't disappear into the hospital laundry. The laundrymaid is you!

Even if you're a Queen among mothers, there are bound to be days when motherhood seems to bring nothing but problems. When the baby's got colic, you've got a cold and the washing machine breaks down, you may feel like taking an overdose of gripewater.

Most starry-eyed mums with no previous experience of caring for babies – and that's 90 per cent of us – look for a miracle to happen after the birth. We expect that, with a little luck and a dollop of good management, we'll turn into serene, super-clean Lady Madonnas, just like those well groomed spotless mums in TV commercials.

What's a Wondermum?

Somewhere on this planet must exist the wondermum. She's that crazy lady in commercials who dresses her kids in white – then sends them out to play in mud because she just *loves* washing. Ever-cooking, ever-lovely, she never gets tired, grizzly, frazzled or short-tempered. It's a wonder that ring of confidence around her perfect white smile doesn't slip down and choke her!

The Perfect Mother, as advertised, is about as real as Mary Poppins and exists only in the imagination of scriptwriters and advertising men.

The current romantic picture of parenthood has been attacked by child care expert Dr. Mia Kellmer Pringle. She thinks it's badly misleading and should be changed. 'Babies should be presented truthfully, warts and all – sometimes fretful, and demanding, often wet, smelly, crying at night and unreasonable – rather than with a permanent, angelic, dimply smile and sunny temper,' she says. Taking the glamour out of parenthood like this won't put off those who truly want to care for children, thinks Dr. Kellmer Pringle. But it may act as a brake on those who have too rosy a picture of parenthood.[1]

There isn't a real mum alive who doesn't at some time feel like screaming at her offspring – and does! Fed up with strained baby food clinging to her clothes, she thinks just one more edition of 'Play School' will crack her self control. No matter how hard she tries, sooner or later every new mum comes down to earth with a bump.

Judy: 'In the first few days after I came home from hospital, you'd have thought I was trying to win some Mother-of-the-Year award. By 8.30 each morning, I was up, dressed and had finished making breakfast for my husband. When the health visitor first called, the baby was sleeping angelically and the house was shining. She looked round and said: "You seem so organised, I can

see I won't have to worry about you". Two weeks
later, she dropped in and found a very different
scene. It was 11 a.m. and I looked the tired wreck
I felt, still in my dressing gown. The house was a
mess and my husband had taken an apple to
work for his breakfast. Everything had just piled
on top of me in my desperate attempts to have a
contented baby, a happy husband and a smooth-
running home. Something had to give so I
relaxed and stopped trying to be a wondermum.'

Too often a new mum has only a vague idea of what's
expected of her. And when she has to cope with a real baby,
she discovers it's not all gurgles at one end but soggy, soiled
nappies at the other, too. That's when she often strikes
troubles with her feelings.

The number one myth of motherhood is that a magic
switch automatically turns an ordinary woman into a
'Mother' the minute she's had a baby. This is known as the
maternal instinct. And a new mum who feels she isn't slipping smoothly into her mothering role may believe she's an
unfeminine failure.

But is there really a maternal instinct? Psychologists say
no, it doesn't exist and that a *man* could have just as much
'maternal instinct' as his wife. When you're new to motherhood it can sometimes take a little while to get to know – and
love – your baby. Like anything else in life, you need to
learn from experiences and mistakes. In fact, looking at your
baby and feeling quite detached from her can be the first
real downer a new mother can feel. One told us: 'I really
expected the baby to be an immediate part of the family,
we'd been so looking forward to her arrival. Yet when I
first looked at her, I saw a stranger. It was only after a few
weeks when I began to know her little ways that I developed
first a fondness and then a great love for her. But no one had
told me I could feel so unmotherly in the beginning and I was
quite depressed about it.'

There are times when you feel very *un*loving towards your

child. Seems like blasphemy? Something you can't even discuss with your man? It's not as rare as you'd think. A tired new mum with a 5-week-old baby remembers phoning her mother in Scotland on a day when everything had gone wrong. Half-desperate, half-jokey, she asked: 'How many years do you get for baby battering?' She told us: 'Of course I would never have harmed my baby but believe me, I can understand why some women can go over the edge. That day he was driving me crazy and I certainly didn't like him much – until the following day.'

Dr. Penelope Leach gives a good example of how to take the strain out of mothering (more, from us, on page 183). She says that the mum who gets up willingly when she hears her baby cry in the night may spend only half an hour feeding the baby before going back to bed warmed by her baby's toothless grin. 'But the mother who fights his demands for food, staying in bed while he howls, getting up crossly to offer boiled water, will end up feeding him. But she'll probably have been awake for two hours and go to bed feeling that motherhood is hell.'[2]

You can prevent a lot of small irritations that drag a new mum down if you've the right attitude to mothering. What's the right attitude? To us, it's a calm, relaxed state of mind. That may sound pious and rather obvious. But remember, relaxation is the link between love and babies. It helps you to blissful love-making (how else can you reach the Big O?). Relaxation exercises are the key to an easier childbirth. And in the same way, you can be a far less anxious mum if you're relaxed. Those breathing exercises you learned for the birth will help your muscles to loosen when you're especially tense. When the baby sleeps, try to catnap. If you can't, lie on the bed doing those breathing exercises, then see how you untense yourself even after a few minutes.

In fact, losing that uptight, downbeat feeling which many new mothers experience, can make you a BabyLove mum!

Help is at Hand

As you're muddling through these first awful days – and
believe us, the first 6 weeks truly are the worst – a neighbour-
hood angel called a health visitor will turn up on your door-
step. You don't need to arrange this. Your local authority
makes it happen, as if by magic, liaising with your hospital.

The health visitor is a registered nurse with special training in babycare. (More about her charms on page 223.)
Don't be embarrassed if she finds you still in your night-
clothes at noon, with housework undone. She's probably
used to far worse sights! First, she may want to see the baby
and where she sleeps to check the room temperature. A
mimimun of 68–70°F (20–21°C) is ideal but it should be
slightly warmer when you're giving a new baby a bath.

If the health visitor asks how you're coping, don't be shy
about confiding in her. Take her advice and don't worry
about showing your inexperience – it's a good way to get the
help you may need. She can suggest a schedule to help avoid
over-tiredness and she'll dish out valuable advice on handling babies. The best suggestion a friend got about her baby
boy was from her health visitor who said: 'Always see that
his willie is pointing downwards, dear. Otherwise, you won't
have a dry eye in the house when you're changing him.'

Every Mum's Biggest Mistake

It was the biggest mistake we both made – miscalculating
the time between feeds. Babies usually settle into a feeding
pattern of meals every four hours. So once you've put the
baby down after feeding, you've got four hours till the next
feed – right? Wrong! It's nearer three. If the baby wakes at,
say, 10 a.m. it takes about 45 minutes to change and feed
your infant. Add another 10 minutes for cuddling time and
you've probably spent nearly an hour. The next feed may
be at 2 p.m. so you've actually got only three hours left, not
four, for the zillion jobs which must be done before the next

feed. If you're on a three-hourly feeding schedule – or even less – you may consider suicide by jumping off your ever-growing mountain of used nappies!

Coping With Visitors

It takes a year to have a baby. Nine months of pregnancy and three months to get over it. But your recovery may be delayed if you've hordes of visitors turning up to see the new baby. You just haven't the energy – or time – to entertain. So try to stall these well-meaning visitors for a few weeks till you get stronger and more organised. Allow only a few close friends or relatives who will visit and offer to help. If some jewel offers to do some ironing or dusting, take our advice: rush to the door and lock it so he or she won't change their minds!

How to get your Baby to sleep all night

The first question every friend asks after you bring your baby home is: 'does she sleep through the night?' Getting an uninterrupted night's sleep is every new mum's main ambition. It means you'll not only feel and look much better, but you'll have the energy to cope with anything the day brings. For a start, say goodbye to a full night's sleep for at least the first few weeks while your baby settles into some kind of routine.

A newborn has no way of knowing that night-time means sleeping time. And don't assume that all young babies do is sleep. Yours could be the exception! There is no rule about how much sleep each baby needs. Just like adults, some need more sleep than others. It's the worn-out parents who are desperate to get some shut-eye. . . .

Letters to a national newspaper[3]:

'My baby boy didn't seem to need as much sleep as other

babies. The only way to get some peace at night, was to harness him in his pram and to let him see me working. I would polish the furniture, do the ironing or even finish some decorating and he was happy. If I tried to sit down to read or knit, he would start crying. I usually had to start working for him at midnight and go on till around 3 a.m. when he would at last fall asleep.'

Mrs. C. A. Dawes, Mill Hill, London.

'I used to have a terrible time getting my baby to sleep through the night. Then I discovered that the sound of a running car engine lulled him into the land of Nod. Now each night at 11 o'clock, I wrap him up soundly, put him in his carry-cot and take him for a 15 minute car ride.'

Mrs. A. Burrows, Eston, Cleveland.

'When our son was a baby we discovered that keeping everything quiet didn't help him to get to sleep but noise soothed him. So if he didn't settle down at night I used the vacuum cleaner. Soon, he would be asleep.'

Mrs. J. Hall, Corby, Northants.

Some wee-small-hour ravers are happy to lie gurgling in their cribs – and you'd be crazy to go in and disturb them. If you're worried about your baby being cold, use a sleeping bag. Or keep the bedclothes in place with plastic blanket pegs. But the babies who need company or food should not be left screaming. A new baby cannot take in a food supply big enough to sustain her through the night. So she wakes up hungry for the first few weeks. But as she grows heavier other things may wake her – like teething troubles or bad dreams. After a few weeks you will learn to recognise your baby's different cries and decide for yourself if the solution is just a lullaby and a few pats on the back; or whether something more is needed.

The important thing to remember is not to jump out of bed at the first whimper. Some babies are restless and go back to sleep of their own accord if left for a few minutes.

Sometimes, a dummy will help a baby to settle down quickly. If that doesn't work, a few ounces of water and a cuddle might help. But of course, if a feed is due, a drink of water won't satisfy her and in that case, give her the feed early.

If you are half-drunk with tiredness, a baby who wakes twice or more each night is hard to take. Especially if irritating friends claim their babies sleep from 6 p.m. to 8.30 a.m. Remember, your baby is different from any other on this planet. And she is living life her way. One day, she'll surprise you by suddenly sleeping through until morning!

When your baby is getting on for a year old, she might start to wake during the night. Perhaps when she was teething she got into the habit of sleeping fretfully. Later, when the teething passed, she decided that it was rather nice to see her mum's face several times during the night. In this case, you have to force yourself to listen to her wails. The first night it happens, you'll swear she cried for a solid three hours. In fact it's more likely to be about 30 to 40 minutes. The second night, the baby will cry for about 20 minutes and by the third or fourth night she ought to have got the message and so sleep right through till morning.

Beating that Tired Feeling

Having a baby then getting into a routine which suits you all takes time. You're probably feeling far more exhausted than you'd ever imagined possible. This isn't the kind of tiredness that a few early nights can solve (even supposing you were able to have them). It will take weeks for your body to be restored to the normal hormone and energy levels. Sometimes, continuing with the iron pills you were given at antenatal clinics will help give you more zip. If you eat regularly and stick to well-balanced, high protein meals (include eggs, meat, fish and cheese and plenty of milk) your stamina may be increased. But here are a few ways to gain more peace and quiet:

Swaddling: If you swaddle your baby – wrap her tightly in

a small, light blanket – you may make her sleep better. The swaddling gives her more security as it is as confining as the womb and almost as warm. Put the little parcel in her crib or carry-cot and cover with another blanket. With luck, she'll sleep soundly until her next feed giving you extra recovery time.

Sling Time: The best way we know to comfort a crying baby and work at the same time is to use a baby sling. For a few pounds, you can keep your child cuddled close to your chest or back. Then you don't have to rush up and down stairs to keep an eye on her which means using less energy during the day. (*Also see* page 208).

Sleeping with your baby: The biggest no-no every new mum used to be warned against, was taking her baby into bed with her. Now child care experts are coming round to the idea. They know there's little risk of smothering a healthy baby in your bed because babies have a natural wriggle reflex which protects them. We've read a lovely story about this in *The Family Bed* by Tina Thevenin. In it, she tells of a 6-week-old baby who was put in the parental bed. His mother went to sleep a few feet away and when she woke, she found that – even at this early age – her baby had wriggled into his favourite position: right up close to her.[4]

Dr. Hugh Jolly feels so strongly that this is the right way to bring up babies that he encourages mothers at the maternity unit at London's Charing Cross Hospital to take their babies into bed with them. The children don't roll out of bed and the wards are much quieter at night because the mothers and babies are happier. (Read more about this on page 198.)

So if your baby won't go to sleep at night, put her into your bed until she does. Then gently put her back into her own crib or cot. This is the BabyLove way to peaceful nights.

The Baby Lie-in

Many doctors think it's better for your baby to sleep on her stomach for many reasons. First, the child gets rid of any excess wind this way. Secondly, it strengthens the back and neck muscles when the baby tries to lift her head. And more important for a tired mum, there's a chance that by compressing her tummy, it can put off – for a little while – the first pangs of hunger. Okay, it's a slight chance but it's worth trying!

There's no danger that the baby will suffocate in the tummy downwards position because she'll be sleeping with her head facing sideways. And if she should bring up some excess milk, there's no chance of her swallowing it and choking. But when the baby is awake, let her spend time on her back and alternate sides so that all parts of her body are exercised.

Cool Rules for Red-Hot Mamas

We believe in cutting corners in housework to spend as much time as possible caring for your new baby. But there's still a surprising amount left to do. If you're going to stay sane, you need some kind of system, a basic framework to build your day around. So here are a few ground rules for those first few terrible weeks:

1 Never put off until tomorrow what you can put off until next week.
2 Never do anything you can persuade, con, sweet-talk or brow-beat someone else into doing. But do your persuading nicely. Remember the old motto: 'You catch more flies with honey than you do with vinegar.'
3 If it smells, wash it. If it doesn't, fling it into the laundry basket for another day when you're feeling more energetic.
4 Do nothing at its proper time. Put nothing in its proper place. Which is to say do everything when and how you want to. If it's easier for you to bath the baby at dawn or let her sleep in the kitchen, go ahead. (And also read the BabyLove Code on page 257.)

CHAPTER SEVENTEEN

Happy Nappy Days

Becoming tops at the bottom business is simpler than you think. Most women still imagine that nappy changing is the least fun part of being a mum. But our nappy know-how takes the nastiness out of this job and saves you money at the same time.

Which Nappies?

In any store's baby-wear department, you'll always find cut-price nappies. But quality really counts when buying nappies because they have to survive at least 2 years tough wash and wear. Terry towelling squares are available in various thicknesses and at many different prices. Take our tip: buy the most expensive you can afford. Remember that the thickest, most fluffy nappies are the most absorbent. And they make your baby the most comfortable, too. The best quality nappies will last longer and retain their absorbency longer than cheaper types. The cheapies will need to be changed more often – so you've more to wash – and they also have a nasty habit of eventually wearing into holes.

Money Saver:

Top brands often sell slightly-flawed nappies as 'seconds'. This means that, though still first-quality in material, they may have some slight defect like drawn threads or the odd snag or two. Sometimes, you won't even be able to see the defect but who cares anyway if they do the job well? And they do. More important, they're sold at reduced prices so they're first-rate value for money.

Nappy Liners

One-way nappy liners are the best thing that ever happened to babies since the safety-locking nappy pin was invented. Mothers bless them too because they make handling soiled nappies so much easier. The baby's motions are neatly caught (well, most times, anyway!) by the liner. All you need is to lift the parcel out, flush it away down the lavatory and you're left with a virtually clean nappy ready to be thrown into the sterilising bucket, for soaking.

Money Saver:

There's no need to throw away liners which are damp but not soiled. Simply put them in the sterilising solution, along with the nappies. Then wash. You can then use them until they get so ragged they fall apart. Using like this, a box of nappy liners lasts twice (or even 3 times) as long.

Disposable Nappies

Some of them aren't. A few types of sewerage systems can't cope with bulky nappies being flushed down lavatories. If you're worried that disposables could block your pipes – even if you shred the nappy first – wrap them and throw in your outside dustbin or burn them outside. It's also a good idea to use a nappy liner inside a disposable nappy. Then all the soiling can be easily removed and shredding the nappy becomes less nasty.

You can also buy disposable nappies complete with water-proof pants, all-in-one but they're pricey and so are only worth buying for travelling or emergencies. Incidentally, putting a disposable inside a towelling nappy is also a good idea to keep your baby drier longer throughout the night. Older babies drink more and sleep longer so they tend to wake with soaking wet nappies. The disposable helps to absorb the damp.

Money Saver:

The bigger the pack, the cheaper the price. Buying a pack of 40 disposables costs less than double the price of 2 packs of 20. As with all your shopping, compare prices throughout your high street and don't be faithful to one particular brand. Special offers at supermarkets and chain stores may often be lower priced than those at chemists. Don't ignore the small, independent chemist either. Because of more lower shop rents and rates, he can sometimes surprise you with a bargain.

Plastic Pants

These prevent puddles on your lap and cut down on your washing load. By saving mums work, they have made us less anxious to force potty training on our children before they're ready. But plastic pants can encourage mums to be lazy about nappy changing. If you seal a baby from waist to thighs tightly in plastic, you could have a nasty case of nappy rash on your hands – especially if you don't change quickly or often enough. See that the pants are roomy enough to allow the air to circulate and the dampness to evaporate.

Plastic pants are designed in different styles for various uses. It's best to buy the soft, pliable and thick plastic type which are a little more expensive than the thin, transparent kind. They last longer, look neater and are softer against babyskin.

Money Saver:

Ideal for newborns, are sheets of plastic waterproofing, shaped to tie around towelling nappies. Unlike normal pants, you can adjust them to fit the waist of even the smallest baby and they don't leave red marks from elastic around waist and thighs. You can buy several pairs in a pack very cheaply. And they should last you for the first 6 months, depending on the size of your baby, though not for overnight use.

Easy Changing

You'll change your baby no less than 2,920 times in the first year. So here's how to work out a slick routine that's easy for you – and the baby. Gather everything you need before you start with the nappy ready-folded in the shape you need. That way you don't leave the wriggly baby lying with her bottom in the cold, waiting while you fold the nappy. You can fold a whole stack of clean nappies while watching TV (some mums even place a liner inside each one). It means you need never take your eyes off the baby because all the work has been done beforehand.

For changing, you'll need: cotton wool balls, paper tissues or lavatory paper; baby lotion or baby oil, soap and water (not necessary for every change); clean nappy and liner; nappy pins. Most new mums like to keep all these together in a pretty basket. One we know adapted an old cutlery basket. The sections for each piece of cutlery came in useful for the baby aids, as well.

Never wake a baby just to change her nappy. We know a nappy maniac who swore her son was positively unhappy whenever he was either wet or dirty. So she used to change him no less than 30 times every day. Honestly! She was right about one thing: the baby definitely was unhappy but not because he hated damp nappies. He took exception to his mother interrupting his rest to change his nappy. So he cried constantly from over-tiredness. Which led her to describe him as a 'difficult' baby. Doctors have found that babies don't actually mind if their nappies are damp or dirty. (*See* page 197 for an interesting experiment about this.)

Babies hate fuss. This is another reason nappy changing should be as swift and painless for both of you as possible. Lay the baby down on the changing mat (cover it with a spare nappy so the surface is nice and warm to lie on). Unpin the

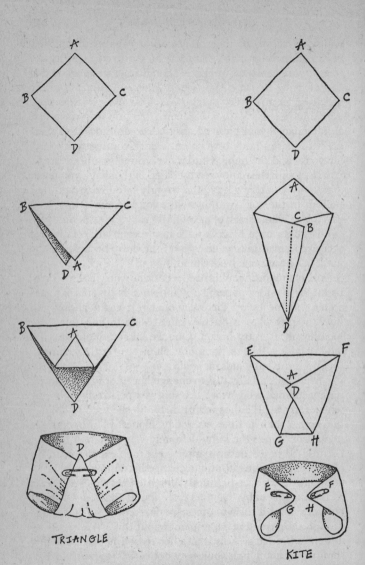

How To Fold Nappies

nappy. Remove the liner. Wipe off any extra soiling with tissues. Put soiled nappy and liner to one side. Then use cotton wool and baby lotion or oil (especially good for nappy rash) to wipe the bottom clean. Soap and water aren't necessary every single time you change a nappy, especially if your baby is bathed and topped-and-tailed daily. Baby lotion or oil is kinder to sensitive bottoms than even mild soap.

Always wipe clean a baby girl's genitals from the vagina down, towards the bottom, to avoid infections of the bowel entering the bladder or vaginal passage. In the same way, don't slide back the foreskin on a boy's penis.

It's also a good idea to leave your baby without a nappy for 10 minutes or so, daily. Babies love the free feel of kicking without a towelling covering around them. Make sure the room is warm and draught-free. This exercise will also keep your baby's skin smooth and infection free.

Washing Nappies

After changing, throw the liner – if it's soiled – down the lavatory and dunk the nappy in a bucket of sterilising liquid. Let it soak for at least 2 hours. Now you'll bless that brewing spoon we advised you to buy (*see* page 89). Its long handle means your hands need never be submerged in the harsh bleach of the sterilising liquid.

Money Saver:

Most sterilising liquids and powders are basically little more than household bleach. So save three-quarters of the money you spend on nappy sterilisers by substituting a bottle of ordinary, household bleach. This does just as good a job and is quite safe to use, especially if you rinse the nappies thoroughly after soaking. An analytical chemist we know confirmed that this was a safe way to sterilise nappies. 'I recommended this to my wife when our 2 children were babies. You just need a couple of capfuls of bleach in a gallon of water. And remember, if your baby's skin shows some reaction, it could have happened using the branded sterilising solutions, as well,' said our chemist. Both of us have used bleach for sterilising nappies for well over a year with no ill effects, either on our babies' bottoms or on the nappies.

After soaking overnight, rinse the nappies in warm water then hang them out to dry. If you have a washing machine, you could save your hands – and make a better job of cleaning nappies. Make sure you have enough for a 9-pound load (which is about 20 nappies).

Money Saver:

Here's how to halve the cost of washing nappies in an automatic washing machine. After rinsing them in clean water, put them in the machine with soap in the dispenser. Then set the machine on 'pre-wash'. This cleans the nappies very well but halves the cost of electricity. On a pre-wash cycle, the water is heated to 40 degrees Fahrenheit and takes about 10 minutes to finish washing. (On the No. 1 cycle, recommended for nappies, the water is heated to 80 degrees and the whole wash can take up to 40 minutes, depending on the machine.) After the pre-wash, reset the machine to the 'Rinse' programme. If you like, add fabric conditioner. In another 10 minutes or so, the nappies will be ready for drying. This is a good time and money saver (we've proved this for over a year, too) but it doesn't skimp on nappy cleanliness providing you've soaked them in a sterilising solution and rinsed first, before putting into the machine.

Drying

Nothing makes a room look more dreary than a great pile of steamy nappies trying to dry. Solve the problem in winter by washing at home but drying at the local launderette. Or buy a drying rack attached to a pulley which draws the nappies up to the ceiling. At least you don't see them while they're drying. More expensive is to buy a tumble drier. It makes the nappies come up soft and fluffy but it eats expensive electricity.

Potty Training?

> When I was a tiny tot
> They took me from my wee wee cot
> And sat me on my wee wee pot
> To see if I would wee wee or not.
> When they could see that I would not
> They took me from my wee wee pot
> And laid me in my wee wee cot
> And then I gave it all I got!
>
> (Anon)

Old wives say that if you hold a baby – even a newborn – over a potty, you're training her to be dry. But some babies who start peeing to order become unreliable later. So all that time and patience on the part of the mother is wasted.

Several surveys which reported on potty training told many a sad story of mums who started the baby at the tender age of 2 weeks but came a cropper later on. Dr. Penelope Leach has worked out an interesting few sums. She says that a mother starting to pot her baby at 6 months, who pots her 6 times a day until the age of 2, will have undressed and dressed the baby 3,276 times. She'll also have been unsuccessful some of the time so the mother will also have had to wash some nappies.

But a mum who starts toilet training at the proper time – from around 18 months – will have washed more nappies but she'll only have potted her baby 1,000 times for the same effect.

CHAPTER EIGHTEEN

How To Make Your Baby Brighter

The staff at the children's home pointed to one little boy banging his head aimlessly against the wall. 'He's backward, almost a vegetable,' they told the visiting doctor. He took one look at the 6-month-old orphan and snorted: 'That kid's not backward. He's bored.'

That little boy was fostered by a neighbour of ours who, expecting a golden-haired dimply angel, was unprepared for the dull-eyed, sallow-faced child she'd been sent. But what wonders she and her husband have done with him. Today, 2 years later, he's as perky, bright-eyed and *normal* as any other boy of his age. Does the doctor give our friend credit for the vast change in the child? Not really. 'She's only being a mum,' he says, 'and all he needed was a mum's love and attention.'

A baby who is stimulated by love, games and conversation grows into an intelligent, alert child. Bored babies whine, cry and irritate. So it makes good sense to see that your baby develops into a warm, sociable and responsive little being. And you can see that it happens to your child simply by giving her not only your love but also your time.

Even at a few days old, babies can distinguish colours and shapes. Mobiles in bright colours and distinctive shapes blowing over the crib or carry-cot can keep her absorbed – and occupied – between sleeps. When she's a few months old, attach a cotton thread from the mobile to her foot and see how quickly she registers the fact that her leg is operating the toy!

If she's a summer baby, you can still interest her when

she's lying in her pram outside. Nursery nurses tell the story of their most peaceful day outing. They wheeled the babies in their prams to a nearby park. With them, they took some woollen, multi-coloured balls which they attached by string to overhanging branches of some trees. These balls – suspended quite low, near the babies' faces – created a lot of interest and amusement among the children. Instead of the normal whines from babies not yet ready to sleep, the nurses listened to chuckles and gurgles as tiny outstretched hands managed to swipe the woollen balls and make them move even more. Try it. We can testify that it works. And indoors, you can have the same lovely result by tying the ball to a thread, then pinning it on the hood of the carry-cot or crib.

Even more important than games is the need to talk to your baby. Start from the moment she's born (even before – *see* page 138). And don't stop. Put aside a special time each day just to talk. It really is that important. Baby care expert Dr. Mia Kellmer Pringle says you should bathe your child in language. She reckons that communication between parents and baby is probably the most crucial factor in stimulating your child's brain. But a torrent of mere words isn't enough. You need to make your conversation rich in adjectives and descriptions: 'Look at this lovely, yellow train.' Children imitate the sounds their parents make – from quite an early age. By 6 months, say experts, babies have even picked up the rhythms of your voices. But they're firm about one thing: just *listening* to adults talking isn't enough to stimulate the baby. And looking at the television or listening to the radio won't improve a child's vocabulary. Babies only grasp language through close relationships with the adults they love.

Stimulating the baby – with colourful surroundings, toys, cuddling and conversation – brings amazing rewards. Happy with her world, she always has plenty to interest her. She knows she isn't isolated from mum, that when she wants attention, she'll get it without hollering. So she has no need to cry. But the baby who's left to cry is the one who's sure to give trouble. To her, the sight of either a pram or a cot, spells

banishment from her mother and she will protest loudly.
And mum will wonder why she has such a 'naughty' baby.

How to Dry the Tears

Babies have only one way to tell us their needs: they cry. And
cry. And cry. Parents find coping with the crying specially
at night, the hardest part of babycare. Constant crying which
you can't stop, can lead in extreme cases to ill treatment of
babies like battering. But dealing with it is easier if you understand that babies always cry for a reason. Not just to annoy
you or 'exercise their lungs'. Enlightened childcare experts
say both these explanations are rubbish.

If you get to the source of the crying and do something
positive about it, the noise stops.

After a few weeks, a mother soon gets to recognise her baby's
different cries and their meanings. The most common is the
hunger cry and that's simple enough to fix – just feed her
immediately. Then, there's the angry cry. That means your
baby is bored and needs you. You may hear this cry when
you've just put her down but she's not ready for sleep yet.
Don't be annoyed by this cry. It could mean you have an
intelligent baby who isn't satisfied to gaze at walls. Solve
this by propping the child in a firm-backed baby chair so she
can watch what you're doing. Or, carry on with your work –
with your baby on your back in a special sling.

The cry of despair is from a baby isolated too much from
her mother and other company. She feels neglected and
unloved. You often hear this cry in children's homes where
busy staff simply don't have the time to give each child
individual attention. But if you're a mother who thinks it
best to leave the baby crying to avoid spoiling her, you could
hear this sound. Run and pick her up if you do. Believe, us
you just *can't* spoil a baby by cuddling, cradling, rocking,
or kissing her. Once again, that baby sling may be the
answer.

The pain cry is unmistakable and urgent. When you hear

it, drop everything and run to find out as fast as possible what's wrong.

Babies seldom cry because they have wet or dirty nappies. Recently, 2 groups of babies were studied when all had soiled their nappies. Half were picked up and changed. The rest were simply picked up, cuddled, then put down again wearing the same nappies. All the babies soon settled and went to sleep again.

Should you Pick up a Crying Baby?

We think you should. Of course, all children must eventually learn that they can't get attention the minute they want it, and that life isn't always so pleasant. But the later in life they learn this, the less painful it is. By picking your baby up when she cries and giving her whatever she needs, you'll make her more contented, so she will actually cry less.

Don't think this is just our opinion. Many doctors back us up with firm research and evidence. Dr. David Harvey, consultant paediatrician at Queen Charlotte's Hospital in London says: 'When some mothers were watched with their crying babies, it was found that those babies who received attention were more content on their first birthday than those who were left to cry miserably. It seems as though women are, in fact, making a rod for their own backs if they leave the baby to cry – which is quite the opposite of what is often said.'[1]

It may seem inconvenient to drop what you're doing and rush to a crying baby. But putting the baby's needs first makes a parent's job easier in the long run. The faster a baby is made content, the faster she stops crying. And the easier your life will be. So if your baby cries, pick her up and try to guess what the trouble is. Maybe she's too hot or cold. Then either put some clothes on or take some off. If she's due for feeding soon, feed her now. Change her. If she still cries, rocking and cuddling usually do wonders. So does singing, while rock music can also send her off to sleep because the strong beat reminds her of the rhythm of your heart. And, once again, at the risk of repeating ourselves, don't forget that sling – the greatest of mother's helps. (*Also see* 'Can you spoil a baby? page 207.)

When to Leave Her to Cry

A very young baby should never be left to cry at any time. But neither should you stand, exhausted, rocking your baby in your arms in the middle of the night. If your baby has been fed and changed but still doesn't settle, you may find you'd enjoy taking your baby into bed with you and your man. Old fashioned baby care experts have always frowned on this, stressing the risks of smothering her (or 'overlying') in your sleep. But Dr. James Partridge, consultant paediatrician of the South Warwickshire Hospital Group disagrees. He says: 'Maybe a newborn would be at risk but I doubt it,' and points out that babies sleep with their mothers in the first days of life in other countries like Africa, Asia and South America.[2]

Dr. Hugh Jolly agrees. He says there is no risk of overlying a healthy baby. 'I must confess that in the early days I used to be concerned that a baby might fall out of bed but this does not happen. The answer being that the baby snuggles up to the mother – not away from her. Watching a mother asleep with her newborn baby, it's possible to see how she lies naturally with her arms and body surrounding the baby in a protective circle.'[3]

In his maternity ward at London's Charing Cross Hospital, Dr. Jolly and staff encourage mothers to take their babies into bed with them. He says he had a delighted response to this from mothers who had 'felt guilty about doing this and did not expect a paediatrician to condone such behaviour'.

Incidentally, Dr. Jolly says when a child has achieved a feeling of security and independence, he will move back into his or her own bed or move in with an older child.

If this idea doesn't appeal to you, we suggest a compromise. Take the baby into bed with you until she drops off to sleep, which shouldn't be long. Then carry her into her own cot. An older child who may not need as much sleep as you, may be pacified with a collection of toys and gadgets inside the cot – with a night light in winter – so that when she wakes, she'll see them and hopefully entertain herself for a while.

Dummies: Problems or Pacifiers?

Babies like comforters more than their parents do. Most think dummies are unhygienic and unsightly, especially if the baby has one stuck in her mouth all day long. But child care experts thinks pacifiers may be necessary when a baby needs extra self-comfort.

Judy:　'I went to the clinic complaining that my daughter just wanted to stay glued to my breast all day and all night. I had no time for anything except feeding her. The health visitor smiled knowingly and said: "Your baby isn't hungry. She just loves the comforting feeling of suckling so give her a dummy". I bought one on my way home and instantly my life was transformed. As a dummy saved my sanity, I say – don't knock 'em.'

Doctors say sucking a dummy may be okay but that a thumb is better. That's because a child can explore her mouth with the thumb at the same time. But some babies are too energetic and fussy to find their thumbs fast enough. For them, a dummy is better than being left to cry.

If a dummy has become your child's crutch against the pressures with which she's learning to live, don't try to take it away from her. If you really loath dummies, there are ways right from the start, to ration the use of one. Tying the dummy to the cot with a short ribbon makes the child connect dummies only with bedtime. Or you could connect the dummy with a loved furry toy for the same effect.

Other soothers like a cuddly teddy bear or a fluffy blanket can also be as comforting as a dummy, especially for an older child. But are these comforters really healthy? Are they signs that your child is insecure? Doctors say no, using comforters is a good sign that your child is developing his capacity for loving. An American doctor, T. Berry Brazelton adds: 'When I make a house visit, it's a pleasure for me to find a dirty, smelly, worn-out animal the child obviously has cared for repeatedly and long.' He thinks parents should show respect for their child's love affair with one special toy, blanket or other comforter and 'for his need of them, as long as he needs them'.[4]

Play Power

Play is your baby's work and toys are her tools of learning. But good toys needn't be pricey. Most babies have fun with simple kitchen gadgets like pegs, wooden spoons and saucepan lids. Crispy paper which crackles when little fingers grab it is always good fun. So are empty yogurt cartons; clean, empty, soft squeezable plastic bottles which can squirt fountains of water over little bodies in the bath. They can also squish air into delighted screwed-up little faces. But whatever toy you have, always remember that your baby's most favourite toy is – you.

Don't give your baby too many toys at once. Her concentration wanders quickly, so keep a few 'new' toys in reserve. Some local libraries have a toy lending scheme where you can borrow toys, then return them as you would a book. If your library doesn't do this, why not organise the scheme among neighbours' or relatives' children? Swapping toys with friends for a month or so, means having a variety of playthings at no extra cost though you should have a compensation agreement among mums should any toy get broken.

Play Safe

Before buying toys, play safe by checking on 10 important points. These points are even more vital when buying from market stalls or at sale time when some stores buy specially cheap job lots to sell.

1 Check that the British Standards Institution Mark (BS 3443) is on the toy.
2 Make certain the maker's name and address is on the toy or its container. (Some foreign firms don't have the high safety standards of British manufacturers.)
3 All painted toys should be marked 'non toxic' or 'lead free'.
4 Avoid toys made of celluloid or other inflammable materials.
5 Check that the toy isn't held together by dangerous nails or wire and that there aren't any jagged metal edges.
6 Limbs and eyes on cuddly toys should be firmly fixed.
7 Make certain that the rattly bits in rattles won't fall out.
8 Clockwork toys should always have their mechanisms covered.
9 Electric toys must always have a transformer if they work off the mains.
10 Ask yourself 3 questions before buying: is it easily broken, safe to be sucked and easy to keep clean?

Choosing the Right Toys

The best toys for any age are those which encourage your child to experiment, to satisfy her curiosity and to develop self-reliance and initiative. That's the advice of the Health Education Council. But with the great range of toys in the shops which should you choose for your baby? Here are some guidelines.

From Birth to Six Months (Eyecatchers):

Soft woollen balls, rubber toys, mobiles, cuddly animals and–
especially important at this age – contact with parents. Your
baby loves to listen to your voice and study your expressions.

6–12 Months (Learning to grasp)

This is the age when babies learn to co-ordinate hand and eye
movements so they love toys they can put in their mouths.
But playtime with parents is still as important as ever.

   Ideal toys include cotton reels, strings of wooden beads,
wooden spoons, tins with stones inside that rattle, music
boxes, nesting blocks and stacking toys, large peg and hole
toys, floating bath toys, tambourines, clothes pegs, rag dolls,
rubber animals, saucepans and boxes for emptying or filling,
plastic nuts and bolts to take apart, books of colourful
pictures, ribbons, box tops, paddling pool, bell with handles.

Sex Differences in Play

Parents tend to be gentler when playing with a girl than with
a boy. Girls get pretty dolls and painted tea sets. Boys are
given sturdy cars and cowboy guns. This is the first time a
child is cast in a definite role: girls do feminine things, boys
get more rough-and-tumble play. But attitudes are changing.
Today, many people think that these roles are the result of the
way society conditions us to think. If you're one of those who
feel that society has changed, you can try to treat your daughters and sons equally when playing with them. Education
writer A. Arnold thinks that parents fear making their daughters into tomboys or turning their sons into effeminate people.
But he says: 'Playing and learning with her father will not
make a girl a tomboy. It'll probably make her more feminine
in the most attractive sense of the word. Cooking, baking,
playing with dolls – unless stressed to an excessive degree –
will not make a boy effeminate in his own or friends' eyes.

They provide a play outlet that he needs and an understanding of his relationship to the opposite sex.'[5]

Keeping Toys Tidy

Three ideas for storing toys:

1　A large shopping bag or basket is easy to carry around the house to whichever room the baby is in.

2　A log basket looks attractive crammed with toys and is useful later for holding wood or maybe, piled high with cushions.

3　Junk shop find: a friend found a cheap and dirty pine croquet box which she stripped and sanded. Underneath the dirt, the wood had a beautiful sheen. She can hardly wait for her child to outgrow toys so she can make it a star feature in the living room.

CHAPTER NINETEEN

Lessons in Loving

All parents hope that the birth of a baby will be the start of a loving relationship that will last for the rest of their lives. But loving, like anything else, needs to be learned – and *you* are your baby's best teacher. For 9 months, she has lived snugly in your warm womb. She has never had to cry for food or comfort because everything she needed was provided automatically by your body. The sound of your voice calmed her. The throbbing of your heart was the rhythm of her life. And the swaying of your belly as you walked, rocked her to sleep.

Then suddenly, she was pushed out into a strange and frightening world. The comforting presence of your body was gone. So your baby cries to be reunited with you, the only safe, reassuring thing she knows. You aren't just her home, you're her world.

It takes more than a few days or even weeks for your baby to get accustomed to the sudden separation from you. The only way to restore the security she knew in the womb is to hold her close. Just *telling* your baby you love her isn't enough. Touch is the only language your baby knows so she must *feel* loved by being cradled, kissed, cuddled, snuggled, hugged, rocked, cherished and caressed.

Cuddle Power

Touch is the most powerful of all our senses. Most grown ups still have lovely memories of babyhood cuddles because they remain deep in our memories all our lives. Being held and hugged in infancy is the first step towards developing into a warm responsive loving adult. None of us can ever get too much sweet smooching, too many beautiful bear hugs or enough nestling in loving arms. So when you snuggle up to the one you love you can thank your own BabyLove mum for the delicious way you respond to affection.

If you haven't guessed by now, we believe that it is nearly impossible to show a baby too much love and tenderness in the first year of life. And it's sad that so many parents hesitate about touching their offspring. A survey by American scientists has revealed how little physical contact there is between some parents and their children.

The survey showed that little girls were touched more often than their brothers but this contact extended mostly to hands, feet, neck and head. Seventy-five per cent of parents rarely touched areas from the chest to knees in girls and from waist to knees in boys.[1]

Parents who hold back don't realise the impact of cuddle power. There's nothing nicer than cuddling your baby when she's naked. It's even better when you're nude as well because skin-on-skin is the best kind of contact for your baby. Physical contact is important for children because the skin and all its sensations are a baby's first contact with the outside world. So help your baby to enjoy the pleasant experience of loving hands by massaging her belly, limbs or back. Make this into a little game at bath time. Tickle your baby so she squeals with pleasure. Kiss her smooth bottom and belly button. And wrap her in a soft, fluffy towel when you dry her so that you massage her body through the folds of the towel. All this adds to a baby's enjoyment of touch and closeness to a parent.

Cuddle power is just beginning to be recognised by scientists as one of the world's great influences for good. In fact, they've found we just can't live without it. Cuddles can be even more important to the development of a baby than food as American psychologist Dr. Harry Harlow has demonstrated, in his classic study of baby monkeys.

He put 8 little monkeys in 8 separate cages. In each cage,

were 2 mother symbols made of wire. In half the cages one had a teat through which the monkeys could suck milk. The other was covered with a soft terry towelling but had no teat. In the remaining 4 cages, the cloth-covered mother also had a teat. All the monkeys got proper nourishment and put on weight. But Dr. Harlow noticed that the monkeys who drank from the wire 'mother' rushed straight back to their cloth mother after feeding. This suggested to him that animals are born with a strong need for close physical comfort. They are not simply interested in mothers as a source of food.

The love and admiration a baby gets from her parents helps her to develop self-confidence and pride in herself. Praise and encouragement each time she tries something new like clapping hands, also helps a baby develop physically. In fact babies need this attention: research shows that babies in children's homes who do not get enough individual attention are slower at all the babies' milestones like talking, walking and feeding themselves.

But you don't need any child care expert to advise you if you just look at the world through a baby's eyes. A helpless newborn forms an impression of the world from the loving care she gets from birth. If the people around her always put her needs first, she'll begin to feel secure, contented and loved. She realises she can depend on these loving people and this trust soon turns to love. In fact, it's a rewarding experience for all of them because parents and baby fall in love.

Around 6 weeks old, a baby smiles for the first time. The parents are delighted and smile back. The baby copies them. Soon she greets them each time they appear with smiles and gurgles. Pleased with this reaction, the parents give their baby hugs and kisses. In this way, the baby learns that pleasing her mother and father makes them love her even more. Parent love flows in two directions. By giving their baby love, they receive more in return.

Can You Spoil a Baby?

Mothers love cuddling their babies and babies love being cuddled. It's a satisfying, happy feeling for both of them. So when a baby cries, a mother's first instinct is to pick her up and comfort her. But when well-meaning friends or relatives see this, they often say that this will spoil the baby. 'Let her cry,' they'll say, 'it's good exercise for the lungs. Don't let the baby think you'll jump every time she cries.'

As a new mum, you may never have had contact with new babies before, and these are experienced mothers. No one wants a spoiled baby on their hands – so you listen and then hesitate to pour out all the love you have to give your baby. You become confused and wonder what's really best to do. A woman writing to a national newspaper summed up this uncertainty when she wrote: 'It's 2 a.m. I get up to feed my 6-month-old son. I can feed him, play with him and cuddle him without being accused of spoiling him and making him a softie. And then, adorable, warm and happy, he falls alseep in my arms.'[2]

Dr. Hugh Jolly says: 'I'm always surprised how often I'm asked whether or not a mother should leave her baby to cry. The fact that the question is asked at all makes me feel that the rigid Victorian attitude that you might "spoil" your baby is far too much with us still.'[3]

And Dr. Penelope Leach who studied the development and upbringing of children for the Medical Research Council adds that because we know babies stop crying when they're picked up, some parents think their baby cries to *be* picked up. This kind of reasoning is impossible for him for many months to come. 'He cannot say to himself: "If I cry and go on crying, she will come and pick me up",' says Dr. Leach.[4]

The fear of spoiling a baby much under 12 months dates back to the days before we had means of scientifically studying the behaviour of children, according to American child care expert Dr. Fitzhugh Dodson. 'At 2 or 3 or even 9 months is far too early to begin teaching him that he cannot have his way all the time.' Of course your child has to learn that lesson but don't try such discipline in the first year of life. Dr. Dodson reckons you just can't spoil a baby under a year old. And he advises the best thing that can happen to any baby is to have her needs attended to quickly. If you can meet those needs – even anticipating them – your baby will become less demanding, more contented and you'll have an easier life.[5]

So what happens if your baby cries and you know she's just been fed, cuddled and changed? Pick her up anyway – she may just be lonely for you. If you're busy, a well-travelled colleague suggests a practical solution. She says: 'When I was in Africa I never ever heard a baby cry. I'm sure this is because African babies are never parted from their mothers. While she works, they usually ride in a blanket tied on her back. With stomach and chest pressed against the mother's body they get constant comfort and security while she works undisturbed. And they're happily rocked to sleep by the rhythm of her movements.'

In the Western World, you can get this same effect by using a baby sling. They're available throughout the country and you can buy one especially suitable for newborns. Pop the baby in it, strapped to your front or back and carry on working normally. Meanwhile, cosy and content, your baby can gaze out at the world or doze off to sleep.

There is a danger that a child who's denied mother love grows up insecure and clinging, long after other children learn independence. This is the view of Professor Ronald Illingworth, the noted British authority on babies and young children. He adds: 'It is well known that mothers who are most careful to avoid spoiling their children are often the possessors of children who are horribly spoiled and insecure.'[6]

To us, 'spoiling' a baby means ruining her chances for normal happiness. If the people who surround a baby in infancy are unkind, rough and selfish, she'll grow up to be like them. American poet Dorothy Law Nolte has written a poem which sums up our thoughts with beautiful simplicity:

CHILDREN LEARN WHAT THEY LIVE

*If a child lives with criticism
He learns to condemn.*

*If a child lives with hostility
He learns to fight.*

*If a child lives with ridicule
He learns to be shy.*

*If a child lives with shame
He learns to feel guilty.*

*If a child lives with tolerance
He learns to be patient.*

*If a child lives with encouragement
He learns confidence.*

*If a child lives with praise
He learns to appreciate.*

*If a child lives with fairness
He learns justice.*

*If a child lives with security
He learns to have faith.*

*If a child lives with approval
He learns to like himself.*

*If a child lives with acceptance and friendship
He learns to find love in the world.*

This poem is backed up by research. The National Children's Bureau in Britain, shows that children of mothers battered by their husbands, grow up violent and may become child-batterers themselves. But loved children become loving parents. So never have a family row in front of a baby, no matter how young she is. Babies are like blotting paper – they absorb every experience which touches them. Even if they're not alarmed by loud arguments and shouting, they may come to accept this as normal behaviour. Even worse, they'll become argumentative and aggressive adults.

If you don't believe that babies naturally imitate adults, try poking your tongue out at a baby aged around 4 to 8 weeks old. The baby will soon open her mouth and wiggle her tongue back at you!

So a child's later happiness in life, whether or not she forms successful relationships with the opposite sex, marries and becomes a good parent largely on her parents' example. And not only on their individual behaviour but on the way they behave towards each other. So lessons in loving and even the baby's sex education start from birth.

Babies and Sex

When a baby discovers her toes, parents smile approvingly and think it sweet. But when the same child plays with sex organs they're horrified. But doctors say that this kind of sexual pleasure is a normal development in a young child. So it's just as natural for your baby boy to twiddle his penis or a girl to stroke her vulva as it is for either to grasp a rattle.

Experts say you should just ignore this activity and don't react either when a baby pinches your nipples or grabs daddy in the bath. But if this sex play really upsets you, gently try to distract the baby with a toy. A calm response to what each child does naturally, is important for giving children a healthy attitude to their bodies. Even more important, it will help to avoid any future sexual hang-ups.

CHAPTER TWENTY

Slim and Slinky Again

Doctors at a London hospital are still talking about a lively television lady we know. A few minutes after her 7-lb. daughter was born, she sat up in the delivery room and asked: 'How long before I can make love again?' With an absolutely straight face, the midwife replied: 'I think it's best to wait for the afterbirth, dear.'

Not all women are as eager as our friend! Especially when some doctors suggest waiting 6 weeks after childbirth before re-starting your love life. But the Health Education Council frowns on doctors with this rigid attitude: 'They know perfectly well that few loving couples could last so long without making love.' Now medical advice is that women should be sure all stitches have healed – if they have any – and that all vaginal flow has stopped, before trying intercourse again. This is usually 2 to 3 weeks after a birth.

But how can you suddenly turn on that old magic tingle when you're absolutely exhausted from broken nights with the baby? If you want to make your man feel as important to you as ever, even though the baby is taking up all your time, take our tip: let your love life swing *slowly* back into gear. (This chapter gives you some help, we hope.)

When you've lost that Loving Feeling

A new mum may find that lovemaking is the last thing on her mind at bedtime. The number one turn-off is usually sheer tiredness. It's quite common to feel you've been totally drained body and soul. In a way, you have, because child-birth – even an easy, happy childbirth –is one of life's greatest gear changes. After all, you've not only been through the physical stresses of the last 9 months, you've also changed into a mother, with all the pleasures and problems that brings!

So the first thing you've got to do is get more rest. Impossible with a new baby? Not if you try to plan your schedule a little. Catnap during the day while the baby sleeps. Forget the housework. Your man would rather have a loving lady than a tidy home. Here's just one suggestion for stealing extra time to sleep: when you put your baby down after the evening feed, let your bloke fix his own supper. You go straight to bed.

In this way, you can sneak 3 or 4 hours of sleep in, before the baby wakes again. So after the 10 o'clock feed, you've had some rest and can begin, perhaps, to think of other things.

Beginning your love life again may be something you'd like to postpone indefinitely. But the longer you leave it, the more difficult it becomes. This reminds us of a story we heard in a hospital ward from a second-time mum. 'After my first baby, I kept on putting off the dreaded moment. Each night, when my husband jumped into bed, I found some excuse to stay downstairs. I felt exactly like a virgin again. When I couldn't put it off any longer, I went into the bath-room and spent, what seemed like hours, taking off my make up. Would you believe cleaning your teeth can take 20 minutes? I hoped my old man would fall asleep. But he didn't . . . he was patiently waiting for me. Some time later, I was glad he was!'

Putting off love-making can increase your fears. More seriously, it can be the start of post-natal frigidity, a problem which can wreck some marriages. Always remember that what happens in your mind, is much more important than what happens in bed. Guess what's the chief erogenous zone in your entire body? The brain. Good loving isn't the mechanical mating of two bodies but what you feel about each other. So don't expect to switch on your sex drive right away because if your mind is telling you to hold back, your body just won't be in the right mood.

Let's face it, most women can't help feeling that the passage of a 7 or 8 lb. baby through the birth canal must stretch their innards into a mini-Grand Canyon. So you may be worrying that your vagina has lost its former tightness and be anxious about disappointing your man! You can solve this problem by faithfully doing your post-natal exercises. One particular exercise for your pelvic floor will prove to you that you're back to normal (*see* page 216).

How to find that Loving Feeling

Just start by being affectionate. Don't expect to reach the heights of bliss on the first try. If you're not expecting sky-rockets to celebrate your reunion, the fear of failure is removed, and you'll feel so much more relaxed. So we're not suggesting any mattress acrobatics right away. Necking and heavy petting can still be as much fun now – with a few of your own refinements! – and can just as easily lead to a beautiful finale.

The classic solution for sexual coldness is also a beautiful experience for lovers: massage. If you've never tried, you may not know what magic a bottle of oil (or baby lotion) and loving hands can work. Ordinary massage and erotic massage are two entirely different sensations. The well known American masseur George Downing says that massage helps more than anything else he knows of, to make sex more fulfilling both physically and pyschologically. 'For a couple having difficulties, it can add that critical element of mutual trust and relaxation which formerly was lacking from their physical relationship.'[1]

But erotic massage does not, as you may imagine, mean massaging what Monty Python calls the 'naughty bits'. Instead, it's all about arousing the *entire* body. But how? Well, you start in easy stages. You may like to take a scented bath together. Then dry each other gently with soft fluffy towels. That's a pretty good beginning . . .

How to Massage

First, pour a few drops of baby oil (or lotion) into the palms and warm it by rubbing your hands together. The good thing about massage is that there are no absolute methods. You can invent your own movements. The only tip is to keep your hands as loose and flexible as possible. Mould your hands to fit the contours of the body of your partner. Start on the main areas of tension. Where you go from here is up to you.

Use thumbs to put pressure on especially tense areas like the back of the neck and shoulder blades. Featherlight stroking of the fingertips all over the body will heighten the sexual sensitivity of your partner's body, says George Downing. And only then move to the parts which carry a greater sexual charge. Like the stomach, insides of thighs, buttocks and lower back. Also give plenty of attention to the breasts, armpits, ears, lips, insides of elbows and toes. Or any areas which respond swiftly to those good vibrations from your fingers. After this, you're on your own – and we're sure you don't need any guidance from here!

How often you interrupt the massage for nibbles and nuzzles is up to you. But you'll find that the feeling of being a desirable woman again and not just a hard working mum is delicious. Even the most tired new mum may find an unexpected urge when she and her man play their erotic love games together.

Perhaps the warmth and tenderness of making body contact again may be enough for you without wanting full intercourse. Both of you will enjoy the strange sensation of cuddling really close now that you've lost your baby bulge. When you do feel ready for actual intercourse, you may find that your body no longer has the natural lubrication you took for granted before. Solve this little problem by using petroleum jelly or any other lubricating cream. And don't worry – your natural juices soon come back.

There's a slight chance that you could become pregnant again in the 6 weeks before your post-natal check-up. (That's when doctors like to fit caps or coils.) So if you're not already on a low-dose pill and your man is using a sheath, you'd need extra contraceptive cream just to be on the safe side. (Incidentally, lubricate the sheath as well to make it more comfortable for you.)

Sometimes, a new mum finds frigidity isn't a problem at all. You could be delighted to find that after having a baby, you feel more eager for lovemaking than ever before. Doctors explain this phenomenon like this: 'All your body's energy is concentrated in your pelvic area to deliver the baby. So your blood circulation surges to that central point like a giant traffic jam. This congestion remains for several weeks after the birth. But the pressure of it while it remains makes you feel very sexy. (Some new mums are delighted to discover they're able to have multiple orgasms!)

Post-Natal Check-Up

Six weeks after your baby is born, you'll go back to your ante-natal clinic for the last time. This post-natal check-up usually doesn't take long. There is a gentle internal examination when the doctor checks to see if your womb has gone back to its normal size and is in the right position. He'll also see if the pelvic muscles have returned to normal. (That's where it will show if you've neglected your pelvic floor exercises – see page 216.) The whole examination shows how well you've learned to tighten up inside.

Girth Control

A flabby figure after childbirth is enough to give any girl the post-baby blues. Nothing is more depressing than being unable to zip into pre-pregnancy clothes. Regaining your figure is not such a problem if you breast feed. It's one of the nicest ways we know to burn up calories. But most mums still don't breast feed and they're not helped by stodgy hospital food. Diet control alone, though important, won't banish those extra inches. If you ever want to hit the beach in a bikini again, you *must* exercise.

Pregnancy stretches and distends the tummy muscles and thickens the waistline. But tightening up this slack area around your middle doesn't have to mean strenuous gymnastics. We know that tired new mums have little energy left for any extra exertion. So we asked physiotherapist Margaret Polden for an easier way to regain a slinky shape. For 20 years, Margaret has been helping new mothers with this problem and she's now the Senior Obstetric Physiotherapist at London's Royal Free Hospital.

Margaret told us: 'A new mum is just too busy and too exhausted to keep doing a lot of exercises. So I've whittled down the usual list to just 4 essential ones. The most important of these is the pelvic floor exercise. Even if you forgot to do the other 3, please remember this one. It's not designed to improve your figure, as much as your sex life.'

The pelvic floor is the band of muscles around the vagina and anus which support the womb and other reproductive organs. When the baby is born, these muscles become stretched and slack. But you can get them back to normal quite simply with Margaret's number one exercise. Better still, you can do this exercise anywhere at any time – while feeding the baby or waiting at the supermarket checkout!

Slinky Sexercises

1 Imagine you have a tampon that's falling out. Try to hold it in by tightening the muscles of the pelvic floor and draw them up inside your body. Gradually pull the imaginary tampon higher and higher, then relax. Repeat this exercise every time you think of it. As many

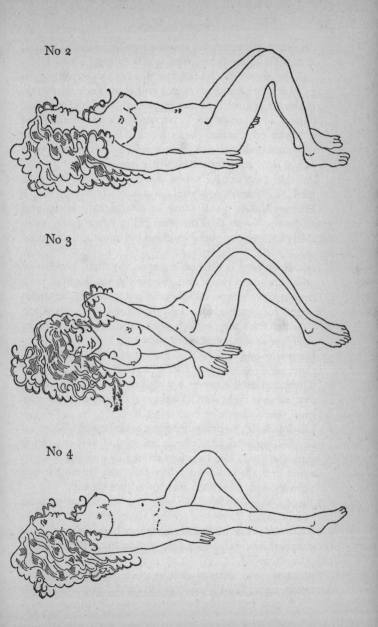

No 2

No 3

No 4

times a day as you can. It's not only helpful to new mums, it benefits any woman who wants to keep a youthfully tight vagina. You can test the effect of this exercise. Just put a finger into your vaginal entrance. Then, as you do the exercise, feel how the muscles tighten around your finger. You can also try to stop suddenly in the middle of a pee by contracting these muscles. If you can stop the flow and hold it back before releasing it again, your pelvic floor muscles are working beautifully. So, if you feel that your sex life is not as enjoyable since you gave birth, this exercise is vital.

Exercises Nos. 2, 3 and 4 tone up abdominal muscles and also firm up flabby skin on your belly. After doing these regularly for 6 weeks, you should have a smooth, flat tummy again, says Marge Polden.

2 Lie down on a bed or on a rug on the floor. Bend your knees and place your arms by your sides. Tighten your tummy muscles and pull them in until you feel they must be touching your spine. Hold them in as you count up to 5 *slowly*. Gradually, as each week passes, hold the muscles in longer as you count up to 10 or 20.

3 Lie on the bed or floor with knees bent. First, swing your right hand over to your left hip until it touches the floor. Then, repeat the exercise with your left hand crossing over to your right side. Continue this cross-over exercise until you feel you've had enough.

4 Lie down with right leg bent, the other straight. Keeping the left leg straight, draw it up so that you shorten it from the hip. Then lengthen the leg by pushing it down again from the hip. Switch legs, this time straighten your right leg and draw it up and down from the hip.

Marge Polden adds: 'The way you stand and sit is as important as the way you exercise. Remember, you have to get rid of the pregnant woman's stance: belly forward, hips tilted outwards. So stand straight with buttocks in and pelvis tilted backwards.'

She advises you never to exercise when you feel exhausted. And comments: 'You'll avoid strain on the ligaments of the spine, which have softened and stretched during pregnancy if you always bend your knees in the exercises, as directed.'

Another tip from Margaret: 'Always place a pillow in the small of your back while breast feeding to avoid backache (the curse of new mums). And never feed the baby while sitting on the side of your bed either with breast or bottle for the same reason. Your shoulders will automatically slump forward and your spine will curve. After 20 minutes or even less, you'll feel like an arthritic old lady. If you must breast feed in bed, lie down with the baby in the crook of your arm. This way you'd get a rest while you feed. But be careful not to fall asleep.'

CHAPTER TWENTY-ONE

How the State Helps

As a lady in waiting, you get special treatment from the government. If you're working while waiting, you have additional rights, now. No longer can you be sacked, for example, just because of your condition. The Employment Protection Act means you can claim 6 weeks' maternity pay at 90 per cent of your normal basic pay. And you also have the right to return to your old job (or one of a similar status) 29 weeks after your baby's birth. There is also a maternity grant plus 18 weeks' maternity allowance. All of which means the State seems to be on the side of motherhood.

But there are a few snags – as maybe you'd expect. You can be sacked if you've been in your job less than 6 months; or if you work less than 21 hours a week, unless by the eleventh week before your baby is due to be born, you've been in the job at least 2 years. So you should have been working for your employer for at least 18 months before getting pregnant.

There are other conditions, too; you may not get maternity pay if you leave your job before the eleventh week. Or if you don't tell your boss that you intend taking maternity leave at least 3 weeks before stopping work. And you'll have no right to get your job back unless you follow all the conditions and also notify your boss at least 7 days before returning to work.[1]

To claim your rightful benefits, here is a time chart which will help. Mark the vital dates on a calendar. Remember, this chart only applies if you are in full time work, paying full National Insurance contributions. You may still claim *some* entitlements even if you don't work or pay full contributions.

It just depends on your husband's contributions. To make sure, check at your local Department of Health and Social Security.

Week 1: Calculate this from the first day of your last period. Your baby officially, is due 40 weeks from this one. If you have been with your employer at least 18 months by now, you should qualify for maternity pay and reinstatement in your job afterwards.

When the doctor confirms you are expecting a baby, he will give you a form FW8. This allows the expectant mum to obtain free National Health prescriptions, dental treatment and, if applicable, welfare foods (vitamin tablets, free milk). You receive this if your income falls below a certain level, or you already receive supplementary benefit or Family Income Supplement. If you think you are eligible, ask your clinic or midwife how to claim.

Week 25: Write to your employer telling him you are going to have a baby if you want to stop work as soon as the law allows (11 weeks before the baby is due). In your letter, state that you wish to return within 29 weeks of the baby's birth and wish to claim the statutory maternity pay.

Week 26: Your doctor will give you a Certificate of Expected Confinement needed for claiming maternity benefits and for the employer under the provisions of the Employment Protection Act. When you get this, you can put in your claim for state Maternity Allowance – from November 1977 £14.70 for 14 weeks. Get form BM4 either from your local Social Security office or from your ante-natal clinic.

Week 28: You should stop work at the end of the week. But, if you wish you can carry on working though, you will get maternity pay and the maternity allowance only when you stop working. Remember that maternity pay lasts for six weeks and maternity allowance lasts for 18 weeks.

Week 31: Apply for maternity grant, paid in a lump sum – currently £25. You claim this by completing Form BM4.

Week 34: This is the last week of maternity pay from your employer.

Week 40: Estimated date of your baby's arrival. You are

now entitled to 29 weeks' leave and at least seven weeks' maternity allowance starting from the actual date of the birth. You can also apply for Child Benefit – ask at your local Post Office. Incidentally, if your baby is born mid-week, your maternity allowance could be paid longer if they inform their local D.H.S.S. A sympathetic official told us: 'I suspect that, though we ask mothers to tell us when their baby *actually* arrives, some don't bother and lose a week or two's money.'

Week 46: The State maternity allowance stops this week.

Week 54 (or 12 weeks after the birth): Your last chance to apply for the maternity grant otherwise you'll lose it forever. (Get Form BM4 from your ante-natal clinic or local Department of Health and Social Security office.) But there's no need to claim again if maternity allowance has already been claimed.

Week 67 (or 27 weeks after the birth): Inform your employer by letter that you intend to return to work in a fortnight's time.

Week 69: Go back to work, having made provision at home for someone to look after the baby (*see* Chapter 24).

Protecting your Baby's Health

Every mother wants to protect her children from illness. And the state helps us to do just that in various ways. Local authorities run baby health clinics where you can get free advice and support. You can also buy dried milk and vitamin drops at much lower prices.

Visits aren't compulsory, but they're a good idea, especially if you're a first-time mum and have never handled babies before. It's comforting to know that you can consult their baby experts without an appointment if you're worried about the slightest problem – like colic and crying bouts, and not feel you're wasting anyone's time.

So it's a pity that most mums in Britain visit a clinic only once on average in the first year of a baby's life. Ideally, you should attend at least once a month until your child is a year old. But in the first 3 months, you could have feeding problems or other difficulties which you could easily solve by going to the clinic more often. It's also reassuring to go there if only to have your baby weighed regularly to check that she isn't gaining too much too fast.

Your health visitor will tell you the days and times that your clinic is open. Simply walk in and introduce yourself and your new baby, a week or 10 days after you arrive home from hospital. Around 6 weeks, the clinic doctor will check over the baby and test hip movements, hearing, sight and reflexes. There are other checks at 6 months, a year and then every year after that until your child is 5.

Immunisation

The clinic is also the place where your baby will be vaccinated. It's designed to help the body fight off infection. This is the way it works: a weak strain of a disease is given to the baby, usually by a quick injection in the upper arm or thigh. The child's system reacts by forming anti-bodies to kill off these invading germs. So if your baby is exposed to a disease, her body is prepared to resist it. The anti-bodies in the blood prevent the disease from taking a strong hold. So while she may still catch the illness she'll probably only get a milder form. The main diseases your baby can be vaccinated against are diphtheria, whooping cough, tetanus, polio, measles, German measles and tuberculosis. In Britain, the programme for babies is triple vaccination plus an oral polio dose at about 6, 8 and 12 months. At these times the baby gets a triple innoculation against diphtheria, tetanus, whooping cough and polio. Measles come later, at about 16 months. Many parents think a jab in the arm will prevent their child from ever getting any of these diseases. This isn't so. Both our children caught measles after one was vaccinated against it. 16-months-old Polly had what seemed like a bad reaction to the vaccine. It was actually a mild case of measles.

2 weeks later, 9-months-old Jordan caught a hefty dose, including the red rash and high temperature. We blamed the strawberry yoghurt they shared one day.

To vaccinate or not?

This is a highly controversial subject. Even the doctors are divided. The reason for this is that a growing number of children have suffered severe reactions to the vaccines. These range from minor problems like high temperatures, aches and fretfulness to major damage. Some have continuous screaming bouts, vomiting and convulsions. Others have more permanent injury. More than 281 families in the U.K. claim that their children suffered severe physical handicaps becoming blind, deaf, dumb or epileptic. That may not seem like a large number, but how would you feel if your baby was one of these? Even the government, while saying that permanent damage is rare, admits 'no immunisation procedure is entirely free from ill effects'.

It's difficult for an ordinary parent to decide how valuable a vaccination is, especially when doctors disagree about it. This is because there are no accurate estimates of the dangers available. So nobody really knows and the government refuses to release figures (on the grounds that they would be misleading). In 2 or 3 years we may have a better idea of the risks involved. A Committee on Vaccination and Immunisation has a sub-committee studying whooping cough (medical name pertussis) vaccine. More than 50 per cent of children listed as damaged by the Association of Parents of Vaccine Damaged Children blame whooping cough for their handicaps.[2]

In the meantime what should a concerned parent do? Professor George Dick, a member of the sub-committee holds the view that he would not recommend whooping cough vaccination for 'infants in communities where there is good maternal and medical care'. He believes that the decline in whooping cough cases is a result of better housing and health care rather than vaccination.

Vaccinations are *not* compulsory though your health visitor may strongly recommend them. We think you should consider these facts and discuss them with the baby's father before making a decision.

1 Certain families have medical histories which indicate that vaccinating members would be unsafe. (Any record of convulsions, fits, epilepsy, or any particularly adverse reactions to other vaccines.) So before you sign the consent form, stop and think. Are there any signs in your family that vaccination could be damaging? Check that the baby's father's family history is clear, too.

2 No child with even a mild illness like a cold should be vaccinated.

3 If you decide not to have the whooping cough vaccine, the clinic can arrange for your baby to have just the others – diphtheria and tetanus – in the series, plus of course the oral polio dose.

4 If you still have any doubts about vaccination, talk to your doctor. Then try to decide, between you, the best solution.

Vaccination is the best way to protect your baby's health at present. But if you feel there is even the slightest risk that your baby will have a bad reaction, don't give your consent. If there is nothing in your family histories to give you cause to worry, then go ahead. It is especially important if you plan to travel abroad with the baby, particularly to developing countries, because these have a much higher risk of infection.

CHAPTER TWENTY-TWO

The Beautiful Baby's Diet

Dimpled darlings with plump legs and podgy tums may make their grannies coo. But any sensible mum knows that a fat baby is not a fit baby. Good food habits begin from the time your baby is weaned from milk to a mixed diet. The first meals you give your child set an eating pattern which affects her health all through life because dieticians have recently learned a chilling fact: by the time your child is a year old, her body has developed a certain number of fat cells. Babies who are over-fed will not only have more fat cells, they'll be larger in size. Though you can reduce the fat *content* of these cells by weight watching in adulthood, you can't ever reduce their size or number no matter how hard you diet. So an over-fed baby has a far higher chance of staying an overweight adult.[1] (And remember, there is a direct link between too much weight and a shorter life span.)

The only way to make sure that your child's weight will be easier to control (even if she becomes plump in later life) is by starting her on healthy eating patterns the minute you switch from an all-milk diet.

Most mums in Britain start their babies on a mixed diet far too soon. According to the Department of Health, you shouldn't start your baby on solids until she is 4 to 6 months old. Until then, they recommend that milk alone provides all the nourishment a baby needs plus a daily addition of vitamin drops which are supplied cheaply by the baby clinic.

However there are a few babies, especially the larger ones,

who have an appetite spurt around 3 months. If you find that milk alone is not satisfying your baby's hunger, talk to your health visitor about introducing solids. She will advise you if the time is right and suggest the way to begin.

If your baby is healthy, contented and her weight gain is steady – around 6 ounces or 200 grammes a week – milk is supplying all her needs. But if your child keeps crying for more at the end of a feed and sleeps badly, this may be the signal that she needs more than milk.

Rules for Happy Mealtimes

You can take a spoon to a baby's mouth but you can't make her eat what's on it. If a baby isn't hungry, all your pleading and breast beating won't make her eat. They will only give her hang-ups about food and mealtimes. The trick is to stay cool and not let her see that you care – even if she hasn't eaten for 2 days. You may be tearing out your hair about it, but do it privately where the baby can't see!

Here are a few tips to make your baby a healthy eater:

1 Always give your baby fresh rather than tinned or frozen food whenever you can.

2 Don't inflict your tastes and food fads on your child. You may loathe liver but your baby could love it (unless you screw your face up while feeding her!). Never add salt, pepper, tomato sauce or other flavourings to her food. What seems tasteless to you may be fine for an unspoiled palate.

3 Don't let your baby know that sugar exists. It's pure white and deadly as nutritionist Professor John Yudkin has found. It has absolutely no nutrients, vitamins or minerals. All it does is rot the teeth and make the baby fat. If your baby has never tasted sugar, she'll never cry for sweets.

4 Ban all snacks between meals right from the start. If snacks don't ruin her appetite they will make her fat by tempting her to eat them *plus* all her meals. Stop her

from becoming a nibbler by never giving her biscuits or a rusk to keep her quiet. If she's hungry, give her a piece of fruit or raw carrot.

5 Never nod approvingly and say 'good girl' at the sight of an empty plate. It may encourage the child to eat more than she actually wants. Just accept it when she wants to finish, whatever is left on the plate. Later on, as a slim adult, she'll bless you!

How to Start

A lot of people who should know better advise you to give cereal for your baby's first solid meal. But cereals are mostly starch and may make her fat. It's far better to begin with a vegetable broth or fruit purée (preferably home-made – their recipes are on page 232). Another good starter is the softly boiled yolk of an egg. (Only after 6 months should you add quantities of the white. It is too indigestible, until then, for younger babies.) Other beginner foods: natural yoghurt, raw egg whipped into milk, cottage cheese and egg custard (which hasn't had much sugar put into it).

In the beginning, the food should be soft and mushy without any lumps. Introduce each food in minute quantities and one variety at a time. There's a technique to feeding your baby, too. Sit with the child on your lap with her head and shoulders resting against your body. You should both be comfortable and relaxed. Use a plastic spoon and hold it at the front of the baby's mouth so she learns to suck at the food. (If you put the food at the *back* of her mouth, she may gag and choke.)

Go slowly and gently. If she spits out the food and shows she doesn't like the taste, wait a couple of days and then try her on something else. If the baby likes the food and it does not upset her, give her a little more. It's lovely to watch the expression on the little face as she sucks, swallows and finds she likes it!

Supermarket Meals: Are they as good as Yours?

Home-made foods are more filling than meals in a can because yours contain more bulk. They have richer flavours because factory-produced meals are deliberately bland enough to appeal to as many babies as possible. But you are cooking just for one child, so you can gear the food to her individual tastes.

Nutritionally, there is very little difference between supermarket and home-made meals. But would *you* like to eat tinned meals all the time? There's a sameness about canned baby foods. All the vegetables and chunks of meat are cut to exactly the same size. But in your own kitchen, you can make your own meals as varied as you like. If you're making cauliflower cheese, you can sprinkle extra cheese for a crunchy topping. You can cook vegetables for just a few minutes so they're more chewy. Your home-made meals can produce a greater variety of tastes and textures than canned meals.

Dieticians think that if your baby is fed only on massproduced meals, she could have difficulty later on in adapting to your family's meals. So try, from the beginning, to alternate between home-made and canned foods.

A Mouli food mill or electric blender will be invaluable to prepare baby foods from family meals. We have a neighbour who has proved how easy it is. She says: 'As soon as Marianne started eating solids, I vowed I'd never prepare a meal especially for her. So whatever the rest of the family ate, she did, too – though all mashed up in the blender. She was no trouble to feed, unlike the traumas I had with my other two. Mind you, she was the only 8-month-old whose garlic-laden breath dissuaded people from kissing her!'

We think you should use tinned foods only for emergencies when you haven't had time to cook. If you do buy cans, take a look at the ingredients listed. If the dish is, say, Beef and Onions and beef is listed fifth in the ingredients, the chances are there won't be as much beef as you think. In Britain, the law says manufacturers must list ingredients in order of the

amounts they put in. So what's top of the list is the main
ingredient. Incidentally, manufacturers used to make their
products far sweeter than they needed to. This was to make
them appeal to mothers' taste buds so they'd keep on buying.
Today, the firms are more careful. So don't add extra sugar
or salt or other 'improvements' to the can.

Month by Month Feeding Chart

Use this ONLY as a guide because you know your baby best.
If in doubt, talk to your health visitor.

4 Months

6 a.m.   Breast or bottle feed.
10 a.m.   Fruit purée. Breast or bottle feed.
2 p.m.   Introduce after a week of starting fruit purée:
           Good nourishing broth (or strained broth from
           can or jar).
           Breast or bottle feed. Vitamin drops.
6 p.m.   Breast or bottle feed.
10 p.m.   Breast or bottle feed.

If the baby is thirsty, try her with cooled, boiled water. If
she hates that, add some fruit juice to the water.

5 to 7 Months

The baby begins to change to a breakfast-lunch-tea routine.
She could have dropped the 6 a.m. or 10 p.m. feeds. You can
introduce her to more varieties of food and switch from dried
milk by 6 months, to boiled cow's milk (though you have to
increase the number of vitamin drops when you do this). By
7 months you can give her cow's milk straight from the
fridge. There is no need to warm it, unless you want to.
On Waking: breast or bottle feed. Even if this has been
dropped, give her a drink of boiled water which has been
cooled with fresh orange juice.

Breakfast: Yoghurt (unsweetened). Fruit purée.

Lunch: Any home cooked, mashed up meal: fish, meat, sieved vegetables and gravy. Follow this with pudding or jelly, blancmange, egg custard, or mashed banana or stewed apple with honey. Or raw fruit. Drink of water (cooled, boiled) or fruit juice.

6 p.m.   Breast or bottle feed.

10 p.m.   Breast or bottle feed, if needed.

8 to 12 Months

She's one of the family now. But don't force her into new tastes and textures of food. Let her set the pace. She'll do it gradually. As her teeth come through, she'll like gnawing on rusks, fingers of toast, or a raw apple or carrot. (If you do, don't leave her alone with this as she could choke on too big a piece.)

This is time to let her start to try and feed herself. The results will devastate you because you will find food splashed all around. Place newspapers on the floor, put on an apron and a thick protective bib on the baby. (If you don't *start* trying now, you could find yourself feeding the baby at 2 years old and even after this.) Self-feeding is easier with a specially-designed curved plastic spoon. It's available in most chemists. At 8 months, you don't need to boil water any more. She can have it straight from the tap.

Breakfast: Eggs, scrambled, poached, boiled – whatever the family is having but never fried. Fingers of toast with honey or peanut butter. Cup of milk.

Mid-Morning: Cup of water or fruit juice. Piece of apple or pear if hungry.

Lunch: Minced meat or veg. Or fish with white sauce. Or whatever the family has, minced or cut up small. Pudding: yoghurt, egg custard, stewed apples and custard. Cup of fruit juice or water.

Tea: Cheese on toast. Or hard crust of bread with butter and honey. Fresh fruit like pear, apple or banana. Cup of milk.

Mouthwatering Recipes

When cooking for your family, avoid processed foods like
ham and sausages, etc., which have added nitrates and
nitrites used to cure them. It's always best to avoid adding
chemicals into the body, especially of babies. Also avoid
plastic foods like instant puddings, package sauces for the
same reason. Steam vegetables wherever possible because
this preserves all the essential vitamins.

A busy mum doesn't cook specially for the baby. She
prefers to sieve or liquidise the family meals for her child.
But sometimes, she may want a few recipes for easy, quick
and nourishing dishes to whip up. Make up your mind when
your baby can eat these, by consulting the feeding chart on
page 230.

Toast Fingers:

Cut bread into 'fingers'. Dip in beaten egg. Fry gently in
butter or margarine. Good alternative to boiled egg.

Egg Whisk:

If the baby hates egg, fool her! Whisk a whole egg in her
milk. Or try whisking an egg into mashed potatoes. Either
way, the baby will be having the protein from the egg without
realising it.

Yoghurt Surprise:

To unsweetened, plain yoghurt, add small pieces of fresh
apple, banana or canned peaches or apricots.

Fruit Purée:

Peel and mash any fruit like banana, pear, melon, peach or
plum until smooth. For apple purée, simmer a peeled cored
apple in a little water, until soft. Add ½ teaspoon brown sugar.
Then mash to purée. Cool and serve.

Quick Milk Meals for the Baby Who Won't Eat:

1 glass orange juice; 1 egg; ½ teaspoonful sugar or honey.
Blend or whisk until frothy.

1 glass milk; 1 banana or other fresh fruit; 1 egg; 1 drop
vanilla. Blend or whisk until frothy.

Family Broth:

Fry 1 onion, 2 celery stalks in butter until soft. Stir in
2 ounces flour, gradually add 2 pints chicken stock (use a
stock cube if necessary). Stir constantly. Add any fresh
vegetables you have – carrots, broccoli, mushrooms, leeks,
potatoes, etc. Bring to boil. Then simmer on a low heat for
30 minutes. Remove from heat and liquidise in blender
until all vegetables are puréed. Pour soup back into pan,
reheat and serve to the family (and your baby) with buttered,
crisp slices of bread.

Tomato Treat:

Sieve or blend raw skinned tomatoes. (To skin without fuss,
pour boiling water to cover tomatoes for a few minutes.)
Mix well with grated cheese. Thicken, if you wish, with
small amount of mashed potato.

Cheesy Spinach:

Any lean meat like chicken or lamb. Cook spinach in boiling
water. Chop spinach into small pieces. Mix with spoonful of
chopped, lightly fried onion. Mix with chopped meat and
top with melted cheese or cheese sauce.

Family Chicken:

Buy a boiling fowl (cheaper than roasters). Put in large pan on top of cooker. Add 2 chopped onions, carrots, 2 cups brown rice, chopped celery (as much as you wish), 1 pint water. Add chicken stock, mixed herbs, seasoning. Bring to boil. Then simmer for about 45 minutes. Will feed an army or hungry family of 4. Remove chicken and broth and vegetables and blend for baby. (Do this with any family stew or fish dish.)

Baked Apple:

Core a large apple. Pour honey down the well. Bake until soft. Delicious for family, super for baby.

CHAPTER TWENTY-THREE

See How She Grows

The first smile, first tooth and the first step are the main milestones in a baby's life. She won't remember them. And you'll never forget because nothing is more fascinating than watching your baby grow.

But without realising it, we parents tend to greet each small sign of normal development as confirmation that we've given birth to a wonderchild.

There's only one snag to this beautiful belief – other parents think exactly the same about their kids.

Naturally, you don't like to disillusion them and boast about your child's obvious superiority. But if they don't seem to notice this, any doting mum or dad may be tempted to fish for a compliment.

Val: 'My own mum was thrilled when I was chosen to play Princess Tiny Tot in a school play. But she tried not to show it too much. So she asked the nun-in-charge why I had been chosen. "After all, she's not very pretty," Mum said, confidently expecting to be contradicted. And the nun, who of course couldn't tell a lie, said: "You're right, she's not very pretty, but she has the loudest voice." '

So parental pride can really lead to needless worry. If your baby doesn't have as many teeth as your neighbours' did, at the same stage, it doesn't mean yours is backward. In fact, there's little connection between early crawling, walking and talking and higher intelligence. There's no such thing as *normal* development. Each baby grows at his or her own individual rate. So it's a mistake to compare your child with any other. In the course of a lifetime, what does it matter that your daughter didn't talk until 3 while your cousin's boy chattered away at 9 months? Eventually, all normal babies turn into toddlers. They all grow teeth and start to gabble. (You may even long for the quiet days when your little darling lay silently in her pram unable to do anything but shake a rattle!)

Although the rate at which your baby develops may vary, the natural sequence of progress does not. For example, all healthy babies first learn to smile before they laugh. They can clutch your finger before they can grasp a toy.

The guide (opposite) to the milestones in your baby's life is just a sketchy outline of the sequence of development. Don't worry about how soon your baby progresses from one stage to the next.

The time taken to develop really isn't important. If a baby is 'late' in gaining a particular skill, doctors say it's rarely a matter for concern. What *really* matters is not how advanced a baby, but how happy she is. Your baby won't do anything until she's ready. Development generally depends on an inherited factor – the growth of the central nervous system. This controls the co-ordination of the baby's limbs, speech, sight and hearing. So she won't be able to reach out and cuddle a doll or turn her head towards you until the nerves governing these actions are mature enough. And the rate varies with every child.

Just the same, providing your child with praise and the right toys (*see* page 201) can encourage a child to enjoy reaching each milestone. Cheering her on gives a baby confidence and makes up for the bumps and falls along the way. It can also make the difference between giving up and achieving something that is almost within her reach.

Despite the differences in all kids, a few general rules apply: your baby will normally double her birth weight in the first 6 months. And triple it by the first birthday. At birth, babies can see (well, distinguish light from dark); and prefer bright colours to pastels or greys. And she prefers discs with smiling faces drawn on them to blanks. Around 6 weeks, she will know her mother's face and probably reward you with a smile. But don't forget, if your baby was premature, she will need a few more weeks to catch up.

3 Months

Physical Growth

At 6 weeks, she should be 2–3 lb. heavier than at birth. Babies normally gain 6–8 ounces a week during the first 3 months. Searches for milk when you touch her cheek. Jumps when she hears a loud voice. By 12 weeks, has probably dropped one feed (after midnight). Now has 5 throughout 24 hours. Most mums at this stage are beginning to introduce solid foods though this is not recommended until at least 4 months (*see* Chapter 22). On average, sleeps 16 to 18 hours a day.

What You'll Notice

Holds head well up. Can lift chest off the bed when lying on tummy. Becoming sociable. Smiling often and following you around the room with her eyes. Likes to stare at bright objects like mobiles. By 12 weeks, kicks feet in bath. Can roll from side to back. Will grasp your finger and hold on tightly. Puts everything into mouth. Including fingers. Practises sounds. You may be woken in the morning by baby babblings. Signs of teething – dribbling and gnawing fingers.

6 Months

Physical Growth

Is old enough now to switch to boiled cow's milk. But bottles must still be sterilised. Has 3 meals a day but still needs a daily pinta. May be drinking from a cup. And begin-

ning to pick up pieces of food to feed herself. May try to hold
the feeding spoon. Sleeps about half the 24 hours.

What You'll Notice

Splashes with hands in the bath. Lifts arms to be picked up.
Rolls from tummy on to back. And soon, from back on to
tummy. Turns head towards sound. Sits up without props.
(Could use hands for support.) Complains noisily if an object
is taken away! Knows you're amused at pretend-coughs.
Can raise bottom above head to get into crawling position.
But legs remain straight. Discovers feet. Plays with toes. Can
grasp objects but needs 2 hands. Greets friends with squeals
of delight. Smiles. Laughs. Responds to sociable people.
Enjoys going for walks. Babbles, burbles and giggles. (Girls
may 'talk' more than boys.) Shows definite likes and dislikes.

12 Months

Physical Growth

Gaining 2–3 ounces each week. Eats 3 proper meals a day.
But may still have a bottle at bedtime. Drinks milk from cup.
Should be trying hard to feed herself with spoon. Most need
12 hours sleep a night. Some may still need 2 naps a day. Has
been sitting up unsupported since around 7 months. Now
tries to stand. Or walk, holding furniture for support. Loves
to look at herself in mirror. Picks up small objects with
thumb and forefinger. May have 6 to 8 teeth. Throws things.
Fills and empties containers. May crawl upstairs. May say
a few words like da-da or ma-ma. Understands many more.
Shouts for attention. Shakes head for 'no'. Recognises some
voices. Sings and rocks to music. Will co-operate in
simple nursery rhymes. May wave bye-bye. Sometimes
learns to blow kisses. Clings to mother, sometimes to father
if around often enough. Likes familiar surroundings. May
react badly to holidays, moving house or strangers. Reacts to
approval or disapproval.

Teething

A baby's toothless grin is one of her most endearing features. At birth, all the milk teeth are already in the jaws, and the second or permanent teeth are beginning to form. However, you may not discover the first tooth breaking through until between 5 and 7 months. This usually appears in the front of the lower jaw.

Signs of teething may be noticeable much earlier. The most obvious is non-stop dribbling which may start around 3 months. But it is not unusual for a baby to remain toothless until 12 months or even later.

Teething is a long and sometimes painful process for babies. Some become irritable and have trouble sleeping, and many mums think nappy rashes are more common at this time, though some doctors say they are in no way connected.

It's easy to blame teething for any little upset but if your baby loses her appetite or seems to have a sore throat don't think she will be better when the next tooth comes through. See your doctor.

To relieve the misery babies often feel from swollen gums and other teething discomforts, ask your clinic to recommend a soothing ointment. Give your baby lots of cuddles and some clean, hard teething rings to chew on.

Although milk teeth only last a few years it is still vital to protect them. Decaying teeth which need removal will alter the shape of a young jaw and affect the growth of the permanent teeth. So limit all sticky, sugary foods in your child's diet or, better still, ban them altogether. Never offer a baby tea or coffee or coke drinks or sweet fruit drinks such as blackcurrant juice which may damage teeth even before they appear. The juice sticks to the gums and encourages rapid tooth decay, and don't leave a baby with a propped up bottle in her mouth for a long period. If you want to give your baby lots of Vitamin C make your own fruit juice by squeezing some fresh oranges, or buy bottles of natural unsweetened juice. Dipping comforters or dummies into honey or sugar is also a great way to ruin your baby's smile.

CHAPTER TWENTY-FOUR

Who'll Mind the Baby?

If you need the money or simply want the satisfaction of a job your biggest problem will be finding someone to look after your baby. In spite of the fact that half of all Britain's working women are mums, getting your child into a crèche or finding a reliable babyminder is as chancy as winning on the pools.

The trouble is that employers and successive governments all seem to be confused about working mothers. Though many of us go out to work because we have to, the general attitude still is that a mother's place is at home with her children. So they don't make it very easy for us to find places at crèches or registered babyminders. Maybe this is a hangover from the teaching of John Bowlby, a child psychologist whose theories on child care had a great influence on a generation of parents and their children. His main theory was that the child would have great psychological problems if separated from the mother. People took this to mean that mother and child had to be lashed together and never, ever split up. But Dr. Bowlby has been taken too literally. Even he understood that mothers couldn't be with their children all the time. But he advised mothers that, if they couldn't be there, the next best person was a good mother-substitute.

He's quite right. There's a lot of evidence to prove that children do become very disturbed if they don't have one constant person in their lives – either their mother or an acceptable substitute. But where to find such a jewel? Ideally, you may be able to arrange for a member of your family to help. Unfortunately these days, many families live far away from each other. And most of them will be working themselves – including Granny! For your baby's sake – and your own, too – it is vital to find the right kind of person to mind the baby – someone whom the child will not only get to know but, hopefully, to love as well.

We were lucky and solved the problem in two different ways.

Judy: 'During my maternity leave, I advertised for a qualified nursery nurse who lived locally because I didn't want anyone to live in. I found the right girl though she was expensive. But it was worth it for the baby's health and happiness and my own peace of mind.'

Val: 'I gave up a full time job when I had the baby but I still wanted to work from home. To help me on the days when I need to see people or finish something urgently, I found Madge, a warm, motherly widow whose only son and family had emigrated to Australia. The result has been that she has "adopted" my daughter as an extra grand-child. Madge is a real part of the family and is godmother – officially – too.'

Young babies do need a one-to-one relationship with their mother or mother-substitute. Ideally, this person should be the same throughout the first year of life. It's difficult finding the right person – especially for a baby – when most day nurseries are not equipped nor allowed to take children still on the bottle or wearing nappies. Unfortunately, those who need this help most desperately, will find it most difficult because of the money involved. It's a pity they don't live in Scandinavian countries where every working mother has a choice of day nurseries working the hours she needs, at a price she can afford. The rare British firm who has a crèche on the premises finds that their employees stay away from work far less often and change jobs far less frequently. One employer whose firm started a crèche used to think it was necessary to attract new staff. But he now realises the crèche is vital to keep the staff already there.

These days, more women need and have to work. We believe it is time more employers and local councils provided enough crèches for them to do so. In the industrial areas of our cities, why don't groups of firms split the cost and establish a central crèche to serve all their workers' children? Until that happens, we think you shouldn't compromise about finding help for your baby. If the right person doesn't come along, we think you should postpone going back to work unless it is absolutely essential. At least for the first year of your baby's life, anyway.

If you can't wait, here are a few of the recognised ways to get help to mind the baby while you work:

Living-in Help

If you're lucky enough to be able to afford living-in help, you can choose between a fully qualified nanny, an au pair or a mother's help. There are several specialised agencies which cater for this market – look up their addresses in the Yellow Pages. The right person must impress you with her warmth towards your baby. And, if not a qualified nursery nurse, with her experience and knowledge of babies. If you're in the market for a highly trained nanny, save on agency fees by writing direct to the Norland Nursery Nurses Training School, Denford Park, Hungerford, Berks. Also look in *The Lady* magazine.

Another way to get a live-in helper is by advertising – but make sure you pick the right paper. For example, trendies read *Time Out*, trads like *The Daily Telegraph*. You choose the type you want. *Willing's Press Guide* – your local reference library will have a copy – has all the addresses of all the newspapers and magazines published in Britain.

If you'd prefer a live-out, daily mother's help, use the local newspaper or a local tobacconist's window. Also check with your health visitor who may know someone suitable. So may the local Social Services department and some are quite helpful.

Day Nurseries

These may be run by local authorities or by private companies. Usually, the demand for places is so great, they only take 'priority' cases. These are children of homes where there is sickness, or great hardship. So there is usually a long waiting list for places. There are only about 20,000 day nursery places for the whole of the country. And there are at least 12,000 priority children on the waiting list. But the situation does vary throughout the country and there could be vacancies at your local day nursery if you live in a 'good' area, i.e., one where there is adequate housing and no real poverty. If you don't and are, say, an unmarried mother or have the circumstances you consider to be 'priority', have a chat to your health visitor. If she agrees that you have a case, she could put in a good word for you to convince the local authority to put you on the priority list. And if there's a vacancy at the day nursery, you may be lucky.

To get a place at a private nursery isn't difficult providing there is one in your area and you can afford the fees. But most only take children from the age of 3 which isn't much use for mums who need to work a few months after their babies are born. Find out about private nurseries from your local local Citizens Advice Bureau or health visitor, or your Town Hall.

Childminders

Most working mums with tiny children turn to babyminders. It is estimated that 3 million children spend their day with minders. Most of them are not registered and are, therefore illegal. Many local authorities turn a blind eye because there are not enough registered babyminders. And desperate mothers have no alternative but to leave the children unattended all day at home.

The babyminders who don't register with their local authority aren't necessarily bad. It's just that there are stiff rules for those who mind children – the number of lavatories, people to cook, strict fire regulations and so on. All of these laws are protection for the children. But to comply with them will take money, and that means putting up fees to parents. So unregistered babyminders, whose main attraction is their low fee haven't the funds to compete. Most don't bother; some don't know they should register. Either way, it is always best to avoid unregistered minders. If the choice is living on social security for a year to give your baby your own loving individual attention or leaving her with a bad babyminder, there's no choice.

Good babyminders won't be difficult to find. Chat to other mums at your baby clinic or talk to your health visitor. Before deciding, try to visit a couple of babyminders if you can. Watch the minder with the other children – is she affectionate? Does she talk to them a lot? How many toys are there? Is there a garden or park nearby? Talk to her about the day's routine and see whether her ideas fit in with yours. The more children she has to care for, the less attention each one will get. Again, don't give your baby second best if you can help it. Postpone going back to work if you're worried about the available help you're able to afford. It really is important for your baby to have the same regular person to look after her at least for her first year of life.

Coping with Guilt Feelings

Most working mums have two full-time jobs: one outside the home and one inside. So the reason they work must be good because it's a hard life with little leisure time. You and the baby will be unhappy when you first leave her to go to work. That's only natural. But if you feel guilty all the time, and think you should be with her perhaps you should stop feeling guilty and just give up work. Some mothers are actually better mothers *because* they go out to work. If you're like this, stop feeling guilty and make sure you have the best help you can afford to look after your baby. Then make up for your absence by giving the baby a great deal of attention when you get home (no matter how tired you feel) and at

WHO'LL MIND THE BABY

weekends. Your man will help, too, in making the baby know that she is loved. After all, it's the quality of the attention your baby gets which is important and not merely the number of hours you and your man spend with her.

Babysitters

When you need a break from the baby, make sure you know the babysitter and, just as important, the baby knows the babysitter. The cheapest way to get a babysitter is to establish a rota system among the mums in the area. Instead of money, you exchange points. But if you do use a babysitting agency, check with them that they have followed up the sitter's references. And if you choose a neighbour's child as a sitter, remember you are responsible in law should anything happen to your child if her babysitter is under 16 years of age.

Travelling Babies

Don't become a stay-at-home just because you've had a baby.

Val: 'By the time my daughter was 18 months, she'd been for a holiday in Greece (at 6 months); to South Africa to meet her grandparents (at 11 months) and to Israel (at 18 months). In between we've taken her on long car journeys to the depths of Wales and Norfolk.'

Travelling with a baby means you need to be prepared for anything – just like the Boy Scouts – and you have to plan ahead in a way generals plotting a battle would envy.

Check List for a Journey

It could be a 3 month hike through Afghanistan or just a bus ride for a day trip to your mum, but pack your bag with not only the things you need but with those you think you might.

Always take spare sets of clothes, sweaters, plastic pants and more nappies than your child will need even if she had a sudden bout of diarrhoea. Disposables are best for journeys. So are disposable baby-wipes for sticky faces or dirty bottoms. You'll also need man-sized tissues, cotton wool, baby lotion, polythene bag for rubbish, small towel, extra nappy pins, bottle, equipment for washing and sterilising if necessary. (One blonde we know takes extra dried milk in case she loses the ready-made bottle. And a spare bottle.)

Planning Ahead

If you're on holiday with a young baby, you'll need boiling water for making feeds and sterilising regularly. Don't take chances that the staff at the boarding house by the sea will always co-operate when you want them to. Or that the waiters in the Italian hotel will understand English (and take it from us, it's difficult to mime 'Please can I have some water –not just hot but boiling'.) Rather buy a small, cheap boiling unit sold by many electrical shops. It looks like a pair of mini curling tongs but you plug it in (see you have the correct plug) put it in a jug of cold water and within a short time, it's heated to boiling point.

If you're going on a long journey, it may suit you to get the baby accustomed first to those pre-sterilised, throw-away polythene bottles encased in a white container. They can be expensive but they're worth it for your peace of mind if you need to sterilise in strange places for a long time.

For Long Trips

Arrive well in time to catch the boat or train or plane. This will help you settle both your seat and your blood pressure. Don't forget many cuddly toys which you can bring out one by one over the hours. Always take jars of her favourite food, home made or shop-bought. Some airlines stock baby food but they may not have what your baby likes. And technical delays can make the journey longer so that they run out. Take extra stocks of dried milk, too. Don't rely on the quaint old shop in the Cornish village stocking the brand you need.

It's best to dress the baby in layers of clothing, not just in an all-in-one stretch suit. You can then regulate temperature by taking off or putting on as it gets hotter or colder. In Britain you need to be prepared for any weathers – from snow storms to tropical heat!

Public Transport

Always travel mid-week on buses, trains or coaches so you avoid crush hours. For long journeys it's worth reserving your seat. And for babies under 8 months, a carry-cot is essential because it makes your journey easier.

In Cars

Over 100 children and babies are killed every year because they're in the front seat when accidents happen. So always keep them in the back seat. If you've a baby under 7 months, she should always go in a carry-cot, secured to the back seat with special carry-cot safety straps. Over 7 months and up to 4 years, your child must have her own special car seat.

Val: 'One of my best friends tried to save money on a car seat. She bought one secondhand, which was £10 cheaper than in the shops, with the right British Standards Institution number (BS 3254) and told me "See – buying a new one as you advise isn't absoutely necessary."

'Then she tried to have the seat fitted by a garage. And discovered that two vital straps were missing. It took countless pleading phone calls and, eventually, a trip to the nearest manufacturers' depot to buy the straps. So in the end, she hadn't bought a bargain at all.'

Don't try to economise on this vital safety measure. Don't take chances with improper fitting. Have them professionally fitted. Later on, have child-proof locks on the back doors, too. If all this seems rather finicky, remember it just takes one slight accident to prove the trouble was worth it.

Car Sickness

Avoid it by never giving a baby milk *en route* in a car because the motion of the vehicle will cause the milk to curdle in the stomach and make the child throw up. A bottle of boiled, cooled water flavoured with fruit juice is enough for young babies. When you stop you can feed the baby and wait an hour before going on with the journey. Have plenty of toys to take her mind off the journey. If the travel sickness is particularly bad, speak to your doctor about a mild sedative which can settle a tiny tummy. (Clear the smell of sick from bodies, clothes and car instantly with our sanity saving tip on page 101)'

Have Cot, Will Travel

Folding, travelling cots are fabulously handy but unfortunately expensive. You can solve this by going halves or thirds with neighbours who have babies of similar ages to yours. Buy these cots cheaper from some mail order houses or discount stores.

Or you can use, as a substitute, one of those circular, netted play pens which fold up. They have a soft spongy base and with a blanket and sheet are ideal for the baby to sleep on, at half the cost.

Some travelling cots are sold separately from their mattresses, so save money by going to a shop selling foam rubber. Buy a really thick piece, cut to the size you want, for half the price of the normal mattress.

CHAPTER TWENTY-FIVE

The Sick Baby

The right family doctor for you and your husband may be the wrong one for your baby. When you and the baby are both new to the mothering business, you'll need a doctor you can rely on. The trouble is that you won't know you've got the wrong G.P. until there's an emergency.

We know a young mother of two who got into a panic when her 3-week-old baby boy developed bronchial trouble. He actually stopped breathing for several seconds at a time. So she phoned her doctor and asked him to come as quickly as he could. 'Couldn't you wrap him up warmly and bring him to the surgery tomorrow?' asked the doctor. Only when she insisted, with some heat, did he come and examine the child. But he did have the grace to admit afterwards that it might have been dangerous to wait until the next day. The mother changed her doctor that same week. 'I'd never asked him on a house visit before,' she told us. 'So he must have known I wasn't the hysterical kind. If I lose confidence in a doctor, he's no good for me.'

If you think your doctor isn't ideal, ask some mothers at your local baby clinic to recommend another. They're bound to know a good baby doctor in the area, perhaps in your own group practice.

Doctors can have an intimidating manner. Because they're sometimes over-busy they can be quite brusque. Some medical men give the impression that they're God-like creatures with much the same sort of power over you. So have the questions you want to ask ready in your mind. Be politely persistent and don't be side tracked by a phone call (or anything else) diverting his attention. Don't be put off by thinking he'll consider your questions silly. If you want to know, it's important to you. So get the answers.

If you're worried about when to call the doctor out at night, here is a quick guide: if your baby is sleeping and feeding regularly and has normal bowel motions, you can wait to take her to the surgery the following morning. If your infant doesn't sleep, refuses food, constantly cries and has a runny tummy, contact the doctor at once. You should also contact him immediately for the following: difficulty in breathing, blood in bowel movements, burns, unusual vomiting and any injury which gives you cause for concern.

To help you, here is a quick check list of the main childhood illnesses which can crop up during the first year with some suggestions on how to treat the less serious ones. Our main advice is never to give your baby any medicine or treatment without first checking with your health visitor, doctor or someone experienced whom you really trust.

Problem	Comments
Nappy Rash:	Sore, red bottom occasionally appears on even the best cared for babies. It is caused mainly by damp soiled nappies irritating the skin. Changing nappies often and wiping the bottom with baby lotion or oil instead of soap and water helps. Also applying baby cream such as Zinc and Castor Oil cream helps prevent rashes. It is also a good idea to take off a baby's nappy and allow air to circulate around the bottom. This helps to dry and heal the skin. For nappy rash that shows no sign of improving consult your baby's doctor, who may give you a prescription for an excellent cream which should quickly solve the problem. Metanium ointment cures bad nappy rash quickly.

Cradle Cap: A very high proportion of babies get cradle cap or scurf on the scalp. Washing the hair frequently with soap and water may prevent it, but many babies still get this condition when their hair is washed daily. The traditional way to remove it is rubbing olive oil or baby oil into the scalp. But even more effective is using an anti-dandruff shampoo. Do not use this often as it is rather harsh on the tender skin of a baby's head.

3-Month Colic: If your baby screams before, during and long after her evening feed, she may have 3-month colic. This starts around 9 weeks, usually ends at about 12 weeks. But the intervening 3 weeks can almost bring you to the brink of baby battering.

Doctors once suspected that colic was caused by a new mother's nervous handling of her baby, gall bladder trouble, a blockage in the stomach and a hundred other minor complaints. But more recent thinking indicates that colic could be caused by some babies' immature intestines not working properly. So gases may be trapped in loops of these intestines giving the baby stomach pains.

Nothing really seems to work though massaging the tummy gives some relief. So does rocking the baby face downward on your knees. Some doctors prescribe a drug for colicky babies which is given half an hour before the feed. It seems to reduce some of the discomfort. Other doctors don't believe in medicines for colic and think you should simply ride it out. It's worth asking your own doctor for his opinion about this.

Eyes:

Infected eyes are a common complaint in young babies and children. Usually they occur in connection with a cold. Symptoms are a yellow discharge which sticks to the eyelashes and glues the lids together.

The baby becomes miserable, constantly rubs an infected eye and thereby infects the other. Keep cleaning the eye with boiled cool salted water with clean cotton wool. If the eyes do not clear up after 3 days and the discharge is as thick as ever, ask your doctor for an antibiotic cream to cure the infection.

If you find your baby's eyes get repeated infections go back to your doctor. The baby may have a blocked tear duct.

Coughs:

You may be surprised when your baby coughs quite loudly and clearly at only 4 or 5 months. This is probably just a ploy to get attention. Serious coughing has many causes and should be watched carefully. It usually accompanies a cold. But if your baby is feverish, has difficulty breathing and makes a definite grunting noise as she breathes, call your doctor. In the meantime to help your baby breathe put a vapouriser (buy one at your chemist) in her bedroom close to the cot. If you don't have a vapouriser in an emergency take the baby into a steamy bathroom and run the hot tap. The moist air will help her to breathe more easily. Any difficulty with breathing is potentially dangerous and needs a doctor's urgent attention.

Whooping Cough: If the baby's coughing gets much worse at night, and often causes vomiting bouts, she probably has whooping cough, even if you haven't heard the whoop traditionally connected with the cough. This can be a very critical illness in a baby and must be treated by a doctor urgently.

Measles: A very common disease of early childhood. While it lasts it's a miserable illness which needs careful treatment to avoid complications. Many thousands of children in the U.K. develop severe bronchitis, pneumonia or inflammation of the middle ear as a result of measles. And some have nervous symptoms. Signs are a red rash or spots which may appear on the stomach or behind the ears. Sometimes there is no rash, just a red flushed appearance. Always call your doctor. He can prescribe a medicine to ease the symptoms. And keep the baby in a warm room. Vaccination at 13 months may give your child a mild dose of measles.

Constipation: This is more likely to occur in bottle fed babies. And it means a hard bowel motion or the absence of any motion for a day or more. The reason for constipation may be too few fluids given to a baby in warm weather or too strong a milk mixture. This means that more waste matter has to be excreted and so the baby's motions become harder and more difficult to pass. Mother's milk has a slightly higher sugar content than cow's milk, therefore breast fed babies have softer stools and rarely become constipated. So try adding a little sugar when preparing bottle feeds for your baby. Or give him more orange drinks between feeds. If neither works consult your clinic or doctor as soon as possible. If there is a bowel blockage giving your baby any patent medicine or laxative could be dangerous.

Diarrhoea: Babies often have loose bowel movements, especially breast fed babies. This may be caused by something his mother has taken. Or when being weaned the baby is given too much soft fruit or other food which slightly upsets his bowels. But bottle fed babies also suffer from loose bowels when too much sugar is added to their diet, sometimes when correcting constipation. Persistent or severe diarrhoea should be treated by a doctor without delay.

Gastro-Enteritis: The symptoms are similar to diarrhoea but this is a much more serious condition caused by an infection probably a contamination of the baby's bottle or other feeding equipment. Call your doctor immediately, give the baby drinks of boiled water frequently to avoid dehydration but stop feeds.

Vomiting: Babies often 'sick up' a tiny bit of milk after a feed. Larger amounts often come up when a baby is suffering from wind. Bouncing a baby about or otherwise exciting her after a meal is another cause. Constant vomiting or vomiting accompanied by diarrhoea should be treated by a doctor at once.

Hernia: A hernia or rupture at the navel which

shows up as a small swelling of the navel is very common. If you press the swollen skin it flattens easily. No treatment is necessary and the hernia cures itself if left alone. But if the hernia changes, becomes larger, red or inflamed consult your doctor immediately.

Heat Rash: When a young baby is first taken out into the summer sun and heat her skin must be protected. Unlike an adult's skin it has not grown accustomed to sudden temperature changes and will quickly react to too much heat. You may see tiny red lumps or prickly rash on your baby's legs when first exposed to the sun. Or if the baby is wearing too many clothes on a warm day she may develop a heat rash on the areas with most sweat glands – the face, neck, chest areas. Take off most of her clothes and refresh her skin with a tepid bath. A sprinkle of talcum powder over absolutely dry clean skin will help. So will a dab of calamine lotion.

Colds: A cold is always much more serious in a baby than in older children or adults. This is because colds interfere with a baby's normal breathing. So never allow anyone with a cold near your baby or even in the room where she sleeps. If you have a cold it is probably useless to try to protect her from catching it. She probably became infected before you realised you had a cold. Your baby may be more fretful and unhappy with a cold and have difficulty sleeping because her blocked nose means breathing through the mouth, always difficult for babies. And a runny nose may

mean mucus from the nose trickling down
the back of her throat and causing coughing. Nasal drops will help to clear the nose
and so make breathing easier. Ask your
health visitor or doctor to suggest a soothing
cough linctus.

Croup: When breathing is difficult and your baby
makes a high pitched croaking noise she
probably has croup, a type of laryngitis.
It is caused by inflamed vocal chords swelling and obstructing breathing. Go to your
doctor immediately for help and advice.

Stye: This is a small red swollen lump on an
eyelid, similar to a small boil. It occurs
when the root or hair follicle of an eyelash
is infected. Try to pull out the affected
eyelash which will help the banked up pus
to drain away, then put hot cotton wool
soaked in salted hot water on the eyelid.

CHAPTER TWENTY-SIX

All You Need is Love

Throughout this book, we've kept repeating this thought: meeting the needs of your child – and even anticipating them – will result in a less demanding, more contented baby. So parenthood can be changed from just a tiring routine into something both you and your man can enjoy much more.

This relaxed attitude doesn't mean being sloppy or living in a muddle. It's just a question of sorting out your priorities. Ask yourself what's more important to you. If it's a choice between giving your baby a happy or a hygienic home, what does a little bit of dust matter really? Babies don't notice highly-polished floors or gleaming tiles. But they do notice – and get upset by – tense, tired, worried mums.

So when you just don't have the time (or energy) to be a wonderful mother *and* a super housekeeper, remember the

BABYLOVE CODE

1 Who cares if the nappies go grey in the wash as long as they're pinned on a smooth, healthy bottom?

2 A dirty face and grubby paws are more often signs of a child having fun than an uncaring mum.

3 A baby will never know if you don't iron the cot sheets. But she'll always remember a mum who has time for a lullaby each night.

4 Babies would rather have a piggy-back from dad than any expensive new toy.

5 What you feed your baby's mind is as important as what you put on her plate.

6 If you're worried about what to do, don't listen to any baby expert. Just follow what your heart tells you to do.

At times, you may think you're just not the mothering kind. But remember, nobody knows your man and your baby better than you do. And if they're both happy – and you are too – you must be doing *something* right, even if you're breaking all the so-called rules. In the baby business, there are really no rules. Just your own instinct and feelings, coupled with a dash of mothercraft. But it's important to find your own individual style of mothering. It'll be the best way for you, too, just because it is your own.

We hope this book shows how to link your family with love and reap the rewards that brings: clocking up more sweet kisses from sticky baby faces; more rib-crushing cuddles from your man and more smiles per life-mile. A BabyLove mum gets and gives so much love that if bad times turn up she'll find them easier to face. Remember, all you really need to bring up a happy baby, is love.

And if your baby is made with love, born with love and grows with love, she'll reach out when she's ready to discover a world of love.

NOTES TO CHAPTERS

Chapter One:
1 *Human Sexual Response*, Masters and Johnson, p. 160, Churchill Press
2 Dr. Rosamond Bischoff interviewed, June, 1976
3 *Orgasm and Labour in Primiparae*, Sam Baxter, *Journal of Psychosomatic Research*, Vol. 18, pp. 357 to 360, Pergamon Press

Chapter Two:
1 *Child Care and the Growth of Love*, John Bowlby, p. 15, Pelican Books
2 *How to Parent*, Dr. Fitzhugh Dodson, p. 63, Star Books
3 *The Child's World*, Phyllis Hostler, p. 89, Penguin Books
4 *The Child's World*, Phyllis Hostler, p. 89, Penguin Books
5 *The Sun* newspaper
6 *The Baby Trap*, Ellen Peck, Heinrich Henau Publications, 1973
7 Interviewed, October, 1976
8 *MS Magazine*
9 *Mick Jagger*, Anthony Scaduto, W. H. Allen, 1974
10 Interviewed, October, 1976
11 Interviewed, January, 1977

Chapter Three:
1 *The Birth Of A First Child*, Dana Breen, Tavistock Publications, 1975

Chapter Four:
1 *The Birth Of A First Child*, Dana Breen, Tavistock Publications, 1975
2 *Miscarriage*, (American) Woman's Day, October, 1976

Chapter Five:

1 *The Medical Risks Of Life*, Stephen Lock and Tony Smith, Pelican Books, 1966
2 *Drug Effects On The Fetus*, H. Tuchmann-Duplessis, Adis Press, 1975
3 *Let's Have Healthy Children*, Adelle Davis, Unwin Books, 1968
4 *Pregnancy*, Pan Books Ltd, (Gordon Bourne), 1975

Chapter Six:

1 Lecture to the La Leche League Annual Conference of Gt. Britain by Dr. Kjell Nilson, September, 1976
2 *Human Sexual Response*, Masters and Johnson, p. 165, Churchill Press
3 *The Joy Of Sex*, Edited by Dr. Alex Comfort, Crown Publishers, 1972
4 *The Joy of Sex*, Edited by Dr. Alex Comfort, Crown Publishers, 1972

Chapter Seven:

1 *Human Sexual Response*, Masters and Johnson, p. 160, Churchill Press

Chapter Eleven:

1 *The First Vital Hours*, Dr. Oliver Gillie, *Sunday Times*, October 20, 1974
2 *Immaculate Deception*, Suzanne Arms, San Francisco Book Co., Houghton Mifflin Books, 1975
3 *Immaculate Deception*, Suzanne Arms, San Francisco Book Co., Houghton Mifflin Books, 1975
4 *Reversal of Narcotic Depression in the Neonate by Naloxone*, J. M. Evans, M. I. J. Hogg, W. Rosen, *British Medical Journal*, 1976, 2, 1098–1100
5 '*We Must Think Again*', an interview with Prof. Alex Turnbull by John Stevenson, *Daily Mail*, Wednesday, June 30, 1976

Chapter Twelve:

1 *The First Vital Hours*, Dr. Oliver Gillie, *Sunday Times*, October 20, 1974
2 *The New Childbirth*, Erna Wright, Tandem, 1974

Chapter Thirteen:

1 *Birth Without Violence*, Dr. Frederick Le Boyer, Alfred A. Knopf, 1975

2 Dr. Martin Richard's lecture to the Association of Obstetric Physiotherapists, October 23, 1976, at Royal Free, Hampstead

3 *Oxytocin and Neonatal Jaundice*, p. 818, *British Medical Journal*, October, 1976

Chapter Fifteen:

1 Dr. Hugh Jolly's lecture to the La Leche League Annual Meeting, London, 1976

2 *Women's Wear Daily*, January, 1977

3 *The New Childbirth*, Erna Wright, Tandem, 1974

Chapter Sixteen:

1 *The Needs of Children*, Mia Kellmer Pringle, Hutchinson, 1975

2 *Babyhood*, Penelope Leach

3 *The Sun* Newspaper

4 *The Family Bed*, Tina Thevenin

Chapter Eighteen:

1 *The Baby Book*, Dr. David Harvey, Marshall Cavendish, 1975

2 *Caring For The Baby*, James Partridge, Teach Yourself Books, 1973

3 *Taking Family Life Into The Bedroom*, Dr. Hugh Jolly, *The Times*, November 30, 1976

4 *Pacifiers*, T. Berry Brazelton, Redbook Magazine, October, 1976

5 *Your Child's Play*, Arnold Arnold, p. 25, Pan Books, 1975

Chapter Nineteen:

1 *Parents Magazine*, Mercury House Publications, 1976

2 *The Sun* Newspaper

3 *Book Of Child Care*, Dr. Hugh Jolly, Allen & Unwin, 1975

4 *Babyhood*, Penelope Leach

5 *How To Parent*, Dr. Fitzhugh Dodson, p. 62, Star Books, 1971

6 *Babies and Young Children*, Ronald and Cynthia Illingsworth, Churchill Livingstone, 1969

Chapter Twenty:

1 *The Massage Book*, George Downing, Random House, 1972

Chapter Twenty-one:
1   *Maternity Rights for Working Women*, Jean Coussins
2   *The Vaccine Damage Campaign*, New Scientist, May 20, 1976

Chapter Twenty-two:
1   *Babyhood*, Penelope Leach, p. 71

USEFUL ADDRESSES

(Please enclose a stamped addressed envelope when writing.)

National Childbirth Trust, 9 Queensborough Terrace, London W2 3TB

Family Planning Association, 27–35 Mortimer Street, London W1A 4QW

National Association for Maternity and Child Welfare, Tavistock House North, Tavistock Square, London WC1H 9JG

Pregnancy Advisory Service, 40 Margaret Street, London W1N 7FB

National Marriage Guidance Council, Little Church Street, Rugby

National Council for One Parent Families, 255 Kentish Town Road, London NW5 2LX

Gingerbread (for one parent families), 9 Poland Street, London W1

Scottish Council for Single Parents, 44 Albany Street, Edinburgh

Pre-School Playgroups Association, Alford House, Aveline Street, London SE11 5EJ

National Association for the Welfare of Children in Hospital, Exton House, 7 Exton Street, London SE1 8VE

Patients Association, Suffolk House, Banbury Road, Oxford

The Society to Support Home Confinements, 17 Laburnum Avenue, Durham

Association for Improvements in Maternity Services, 67 Lennard Road, Penge, London, SE20 7LY

National Advisory Centre on Careers for Women, 251 Brompton Road, London SW3 2HB

National Housewives Register (clubs to stop you becoming a cabbage, write for your nearest branch) to the National Organiser, Mrs Marie Price, 3 The Garden, Lower Common, Gilwern, Abergavenny, Gwent

Advisory Centre for Education, 32 Trumpington Street, Cambridge CB2 1QY

Child-minding Research and Development Unit (helps parents and child minders), 32 Trumpington Street, Cambridge

Kindergartens for Commerce, 59 Rectory Road, Beckenham, Kent (will establish a crèche in your firm – so put pressure on employers!)

Nina West Homes (helps single mothers), 12 Hampstead Hill Gardens, London NW3 2PL

Part Time Careers, 10 Golden Square, London W1R 7AF

Singlehanded Ltd. (helps one parent families), 68 Lewes Road, Haywards Heath, Sussex RH17 7FX

The Acupuncturists Association Register Ltd., 34 Alderney Street, London SW1

ADDITIONAL READING

1 *Everywoman* by Derek Llewellyn Jones (Faber and Faber, 1971)

2 *Pregnancy* by Gordon Bourne (Pan, 1975)

3 *The New Childbirth* by Erna Wright (Tandem, 1964)

4 *The Joy of Sex*, edited by Dr. Alex Comfort (Crown Publications, 1972)

5 *Let's Have Healthy Children* by Adelle Davis (Allen & Unwin, 1968)

6 *Babyhood* by Penelope Leach (Pelican, 1975))

7 *The Newborn Baby* (Consumers' Association, 1972)

8 *Pregnancy Month by Month* (Consumers' Association, 1968)

9 *Expectant Fathers* by Betty Parsons (Robert Yeatman, 1975)

10 *Immaculate Deception* by Suzanne Arms (Houghton Mifflin, 1975)

11 *Our Bodies, Our Selves* by Boston Women's Health Book Collective (Simon and Schuster, 1976)

12 *Birth* by Caterine Millinaire (Harmony Books, 1974)

13 *Maternity Rights for Working Women* by Jean Coussins (National Council for Civil Liberties, 1976)

14 *Child Care and the Growth of Love* by John Bowlby (Penguin, 1953)

15 *The Baby Book* by Dr. David Harvey (Marshall Cavendish, 1975)

16 *Understanding Your Child from Birth to Three* by Joseph Church (Wildwood House, 1975)

17 *Your Child's Play* by Arnold Arnold (Pan, 1975)

18 *The Medical Risks of Life* by Stephen Lock and Tony Smith (Pelican, 1976)

19 *Book of Child Care* by Hugh Jolly (Allen & Unwin, 1975)

20 *The Needs of Children* by Mia Kellmer Pringle (Hutchinson Educational, 1975)

21 *Present Day Practice in Infant Feeding* (Government Report chaired by Professor T. Oppè, H.M.S.O., 1974)

22 *The Child's World* by Phyllis Hostler (Penguin, 1965)

23 *Human Sexual Response* by Masters and Johnston (Churchill Press)

24 *The Birth of a First Child* by Dana Breen (Tavistock Publications, 1975)

25 *Caring for the Baby* by James Partridge (Teach Yourself Books, 1973)

26 *Double Shift (for working mothers)* by Barbara Toner (Arrow, 1975)

27 *The Child, The Family and the Outside World* by D. W. Winnicott (Pelican, 1964)

28 *Goodbye Father* by Maureen Green (Routledge & Kegan Paul, 1976)

29 *Understanding Your Baby* by Dorothy Baldwin (Ebury Press, 1976)

30 *Mothers: their Powers and Influence* by Ann Dally (Weidenfeld and Nicholson, 1976)

31 *But What About the Children? (A working parents' guide to child-care)* by Judith Hann (The Bodley Head, 1976)

32 *The Continuum Concept* by Jean Liedloff (Futura Books, 1976)

33 *The Massage Book* by George Downing (Random House, 1972)

34 *Cooking for a Baby* by Sylvia Hull (The Illustration Publications Co Ltd, 1976)

35 *Birth Without Violence* by Dr. Frederick Le Boyer (Alfred A. Knopf, NY, 1975)

Index